NOURISHING
THE
BODY
TEMPLE

NOURISHING THE BODY TEMPLE

by Simone Gabbay, R.N.C.P.

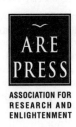

A·R·E PRESS

ASSOCIATION FOR
RESEARCH AND
ENLIGHTENMENT

A.R.E. Press • Virginia Beach • Virginia

A.R.E. Press
215 67th Street
Virginia Beach, VA 23451-2061

Library of Congress Cataloging-in-Publication Data
Gabbay, Simone.
    Nourishing the body temple / by Simone Gabbay.
        p.   cm.
    Includes bibliographical references.
    ISBN 0-87604-423-2
    1. Nutrition.   2. Holistic medicine.   3. Alternative medi-
cine. 4. Food—Therapeutic use. I. Title.
RA784.G32   1999
613.2—dc21   98-56084

A Note to the Reader:

No part of this book is intended to substitute for competent medical
diagnosis, nor does the A.R.E. endorse any of the information contained herein as prescription for the treatment of disease. Edgar
Cayce gave health readings for particular individuals with specific
conditions; therefore, any application of his advice in present-day
diet planning should be undertaken only after consulting with a certified nutrition expert or other professional practitioner in a related
field. It is especially important that you do not discontinue any prescribed diet or treatment without the full concurrence of your doctor.

Cover design by Lightbourne Images

Dedication

This book is dedicated to my husband,
Eliahu, and our son, Benjamin. Their love,
devotion, and encouragement have
nurtured this project to completion.

Contents

Acknowledgments

I would like to express my sincere appreciation to the following individuals who have, in many ways, given their support to this project: Dr. Theodore A. Baroody, Joseph W. Dunn, Elaine Hruska, Chris Jackson, Susan Lendvay, Dr. William A. McGarey, Cathy Merchand, Jon Robertson, A. Robert Smith, Francis B. Sporer, Mark Thurston, and John Van Auken.

Foreword

FOOD HAS SUCH a significant part to play in our lives. Most of us think we need to stop three times a day, bless the food that someone has prepared for us, and know that what we are eating nourishes and heals our bodies. Preparation of food has become a science, and those who cook often become well known and even famous in the practice of their chosen profession.

In the inaugural meeting of the American Holistic Medical Association, it was pointed out by the physician who spoke on nutrition that there are probably as many diets recommended by physicians as there are physicians. We adopt diets to lose weight, diets to gain weight, diets to maintain health, and diets to regain health. Indeed, we are urged to pay attention to all aspects of all that we would put into our mouths.

This book, however, appeals to me more as a guide and resource for anyone who wants to continue learning not only what Cayce had to say about the use of food and secrets that can be utilized in daily life, but also how an enlightened nutritionist has put this knowledge into practice in her professional life. As you read the pages of this book, you will realize how deeply Simone Gabbay has made the Edgar Cayce readings a part of her life, and drawn from them important bits and pieces that bring to our attention the holistic nature that Cayce uses even when dealing with the subject of nutrition.

The importance of alkalinity in the fluids and tissues of the body, for instance, is discussed in chapter 2. The pH balance is always associated with immunity and the body's ability to keep us healthy. When foods are metabolized, they always create either an acid or an alkaline response in the body. You will find a wealth of information here that will help you to choose better how food, selected and prepared in the right way, will have a major influence on your daily health.

In reading through this manuscript, I was reminded of the meal which two of Jesus' disciples shared with the Master in Emmaus. Everything Jesus did was a manifestation of light in this material world, and this event was no exception.

According to Luke's account (Luke 24:13-32), Jesus joined the two disciples on the seven-mile walk from Jerusalem to Emmaus. They didn't recognize Him, however, apparently because He was in His resurrected body. He entered in their discussion about the events of the past three days and told them how all that they were discussing had been predicted by Moses and their own prophets. They wanted to hear more and asked Jesus to remain with them at the inn where they were to stay. He agreed, and when they sat down to eat dinner together, He took bread and blessed it and offered it to them. At that point, their eyes were opened, they recognized Him, and He vanished from their sight.

Ever since I truly recognized the importance of that story, I have felt that sharing a meal is a spiritual event which gives those who take part in it an opportunity to gain soul growth. And, at the same time, the food is enhanced in its ability to make the body healthier in its consumption.

I see this book, then, as a true guide of nutritional information—a resource book—from someone who has not only researched the Cayce readings in addition to more traditional sources, but has put them into action in her life. That makes for truth.

William A. McGarey, M.D.

1

The Cayce Diet:
A Tool for Soul Empowerment

For it is in Him ye live, and move, and have thy being. And it is in thy body-temple where He hath promised to meet thee—in the holy of holies.   1992-1

GOOD NUTRITION IS about selecting the right foods. And how fortunate we are to be able to make such choices. For most of us, food is abundantly available. The shelves in our supermarkets are overflowing with the fruits of the earth, attractively arranged and enticingly presented. Within moderate budgets, we can usually afford to buy what we need. Often our biggest problem is deciding *what* to make for dinner!

The endless lineups at food banks, however, tell a different story. The folks who turn up there cannot be choosy. They just want something to eat. A warm bowl of soup, a sandwich, anything to get rid of that gnawing, hungry feeling. These people are not concerned with counting calories, nor with the carbohydrate-versus-protein debate. Just give them FOOD.

Similarly, the desperate mother in a drought-stricken third-world country who brings her starving child to a feeding station can hardly concern herself with details about the child's vitamin intake. When hunger is the enemy, the question of *whether* there will be food becomes more important than *what* food it should be.

Even Edgar Cayce, who faced his own share of economic uncertainty, did not always know where his next meal would come from or what it would consist of. Yet it is his readings that gave the world an unprecedented source of insights on how food energies interact with body, mind, and spirit to create health or illness.

Do we need to question our priorities then? Is it right for us to be concerned about which foods are good for us, when others have no food at all? The Cayce readings tell us that reasonable concern for diet is not misplaced, because a healthier body allows for a more complete unfoldment of our spiritual potential:

> The diet—as the body sees and understands—is as necessary [an] element as *any* that may be chosen. As the body builds mentally, so may the body build physically by the choice of those foods or valuations from same that will sustain or maintain—within a developing influence *in* the physical forces—that proper relationship between a mental, a spiritual, and even physical forces in same. 1909-2

The task of sustaining the body, through proper nutrition and other measures, thus becomes a *spiritual re-*

sponsibility. It becomes a goal fueled by the sacred purpose of empowering the soul—the God-self of each individual—to more perfectly express and experience the full spectrum of its divine attributes.

Moreover, a healthier body can increase our capacity to serve others, including those threatened by hunger and starvation. Choosing a healthful diet such as the one outlined by Cayce—rich in fruits and vegetables and considerably lower in animal protein than the typical North American fare—may have a more measurable influence on world hunger than is evident: It has been estimated that if Americans were to reduce their meat intake by just 10 percent, the savings of grain (diverted from animal feed) could adequately feed millions of people who would otherwise face starvation.[1]

We might even save some of our own lives: According to a report by the U.S. Surgeon General, diet plays a major role in more than two-thirds of all deaths in the United States. As a steady flow of scientific research results reconfirms almost daily, good nutrition is our first line of defense against physical and mental deterioration, illness, and premature death from degenerative disease. Among the many modalities of natural healing available to us today, the study and application of nutrition is emerging as an increasingly popular self-help method for improving health and well-being.

It is also an appropriate way of expressing our gratitude to the Creative Forces for the wonderful blessings of food.

An Overview of Cayce's Holistic Approach to Nutrition

In the Cayce readings, diet is featured prominently as both a preventative and a therapeutic measure. For nearly every ailment he was asked about, Cayce suggested dietary adjustments, along with other therapies and remedies. Although much of this nutritional advice was offered to individuals with differing biochemical constitutions and specific pathological conditions, there are many common elements which form the basis of what students of the readings have termed *the Cayce diet.*

The Cayce diet represents one of many links in the holistic philosophy of the readings. The word *holistic* is derived from the Greek *holos,* which translates into *whole,* or *complete.* Holistic healing recognizes and honors the essential unity of body, mind, and spirit, as well as the interrelationship between an individual's state of health and his or her environment.

The Cayce readings on diet and health clearly project this philosophy. As important as what we feed the body are the thoughts that we feed the mind. Reading 288-38 gives us the key to this important concept: *"What we think and what we eat—combined together—make what we are, physically and mentally."* The vibrational energy of the food interacts with the mental energy created by our thoughts, and they are both reactive to each other. Together, they create the aspect of our being that represents us in this lifetime upon the earth. With our intentions and actions, we choose to allow certain foods and thoughts to enter our bodies and minds, thereby continuously directing the re-creation of our mental and physical selves. Whether we realize it or not, we are *cocreators* with God, as Cayce tells us in reading 2246-1: *"Thus is each soul, each entity, a cocreator with that universal consciousness ye call God."* With this concept in mind, we can look upon diet as one of the tools available to us in this glorious act of cocreation.

Fruits and Vegetables

Decades before extensive research delivered scientific proof that an increased consumption of fruits and vegetables protects against degenerative disease, the Cayce readings emphasized the importance of a plant-based diet for the maintenance of good health and the prevention of illness. The new Food Guide Pyramid issued by the U.S. Departments of Agriculture and Health and Human Services now recommends an increased number of servings from this important food group. Nevertheless, the proportionate amounts of vegetables recommended in the readings far exceed what the average person was then, and still is, accustomed to consuming.

Fresh vegetables and fruits form the mainstay of the Cayce diet with good reason. They supply an abundance of vitamins and minerals and produce an alkaline reaction after being metabolized in the body. Meats, grains, and other foods high in protein or starch, as well as refined sugar, are acid producing. The readings emphasize the importance of keeping 80 percent of the diet alkalizing to ensure an optimal state of health and to boost the body's immunity to colds and infection.[2] For most of us, this means completely reversing the traditional role of vegetables as a "side dish." In the Cayce diet, meals are built around vegetables and accompanied by small portions of animal protein and limited amounts of grains or other starchy foods.

The types of vegetables most often mentioned in the readings are those belonging to the green leafy and yellow or orange varieties. These colorful vegetables are a virtual storehouse of concentrated nutrients. Nutrition researchers today are just skimming the surface in identifying the powerful phytochemical components which give them their tremendous healing potential.

Green veggies owe their color to chlorophyll, an effective detoxifying and anti-inflammatory agent. Chlorophyll is also one of the best natural sources of magnesium, an important element in the utilization of calcium in the body. In addition, green vegetables supply many other minerals, vitamins, bioflavonoids, and essential fatty acids. Yellow and orange veggies are an excellent source of cancer-fighting carotenoids, as well as the B-complex vitamins and several minerals.

Cayce recommended that the vegetables and fruits in our diet be as field-fresh as possible, since nutrient losses multiply with each day of storage. Modern agricultural methods of premature harvesting, transport, and processing, as well as subsequent cooking, can also adversely affect nutrient content. The following guidelines, drawn from Cayce's recommendations, can help us to maximize nutrient intake by emphasizing fresh, unprocessed foods.

- One meal each day, preferably the noon meal, should be based on fresh and raw vegetables, such as leaf lettuce, carrots, celery, peppers, radishes, onions, sprouts, and tomatoes (in season), prepared as a salad. Occasionally, a raw fruit salad may be substituted for the vegetables.
- To minimize nutrient losses when cooking vegetables, the preferred methods are steaming or cooking in Patapar paper, a vegetable parchment.[3]
- Whenever possible, it is best to select locally grown fruits and vegetables in season.

Grains, Legumes, and Nuts

Grains. The increasing popularity of whole-grain products in recent years bears witness to a growing health consciousness among consumers. Edgar Cayce frequently suggested that whole grains be incorporated into the diet, either in the form of whole-wheat bread or as a well-cooked cereal at breakfast. Whole grains are high in fiber, and they supply a number of important vitamins (especially E and B complex and minerals such as iron, chromium, and manganese).

The readings emphasize, however, that cereals should never be combined at the same meal with citrus fruits or their juices, although these are highly recommended as breakfast foods at other times. The exception is whole-wheat bread in small amounts, which is considered to be compatible with citrus juice in most cases.

Legumes. Dried peas, beans, and lentils are rich in B vitamins and several minerals. Particularly when combined with a whole grain to complement the full range of essential amino acids, they are a good source of protein often relied on by vegetarians. However, they are difficult to digest, especially if not properly prepared. Cayce recommended legumes for their high nutritional value, but he cautioned that they should be consumed in small amounts and that each pod vegetable should always be balanced with at least one leafy (and nonstarchy) vegetable.

Nuts. Nuts, especially almonds, are frequently recommended for their strengthening qualities. The readings even suggest that eating a few almonds daily will provide anticarcinogenic protection. Almonds are high in fiber and contain several important minerals, amino compounds, and vitamins, notably B and E.

Animal Protein, Fats, and Oils

Meats and Fish. Fish, fowl, and lamb are the flesh foods most often featured in the Cayce diet, usually to complement an evening meal of cooked or steamed vegetables. Meat and fish should be consumed in small quantities and should never be fried, but rather roasted,

baked, or broiled. Eating red meat is not generally recommended. However, wild game, including rabbit and
squirrel meats, as well as organ meats, such as liver, kidney, and brain, are sometimes recommended for their
nerve- and blood-building qualities. In some cases,
small amounts of juice extracted from meats through
heat are said to be preferable to the flesh itself. Beef juice,
in particular, is considered to have medicinal value and
strengthening properties and is especially recommended for those who are ill or convalescing. Pork is to
be avoided, with the exception of a little crisp bacon at
breakfast occasionally. (It is interesting to note that in a
recent study conducted by the Karmanos Cancer Institute, at Wayne State University in Detroit, high beef and
pork consumption was identified as a risk factor for
greater DNA damage related to breast cancer.)

Eggs. Eggs, preferably soft boiled, are often recommended for the breakfast meal. In many cases, Cayce
preferred that only the yolk be eaten, since egg whites
are difficult to digest. Egg yolks, particularly those from
eggs laid by grain-fed, free-range hens, contain valuable
nutrients, including protein, vitamins A, B, D, and E,
phosphorus, iron, and essential fatty acids. They are also
an excellent source of lecithin, a phospholipid that promotes the synthesis of cholesterol. A substance often
misunderstood today, cholesterol acts as a disease-fight-
ing antioxidant and is a precursor to important hormones, bile salts, and vitamin D. Research has shown
that dietary intake of cholesterol has little or no effect on
cholesterol circulating in the blood. High levels of serum
cholesterol are not the *cause* of heart disease, but rather
one of its indicators, since cholesterol lines the blood
vessels to protect them against further damage. We need
not fear egg yolks, nor other sources of dietary cholesterol, unless the cholesterol is oxidized through exposure to air and excessive heat, such as occurs when an

egg is fried or scrambled. Cayce's recommendation to eat eggs that have been "coddled" (soft-boiled) is the perfect solution for benefiting from the egg's considerable nutritional potential without risking oxidation of the cholesterol in the yolk.

Milk. In the way of milk products, the readings mostly favor raw milk, or fermented milk products such as buttermilk or yogurt. Good-quality raw milk is difficult to obtain nowadays, leaving the consumer with the poor choice of pasteurized, homogenized milk, usually from cows fed antibiotics and hormones to increase milk production. Many people, especially those who are lactose-intolerant, do better with dairy products fermented with lactic-acid bacteria, because the milk protein and fat are predigested. Extensive research has shown that fermented milk products such as yogurt offer considerable health benefits, primarily by promoting the colonization of "friendly" bacteria in the intestinal tract.

Cheese. The readings recommend that cheeses be eaten in moderation; and soft types of cheese are preferred. Eating cheese at the same meal as other protein foods, or combining cheese with quantities of starches, is advised against. In general, high-protein and high-starch foods should not be combined in the same meal, because their digestion requires different gastric secretions.

Butter. The Cayce diet permits the use of moderate amounts of butter, spread on whole-wheat toast or dotted on cooked vegetables. As with eggs, the popular notion that butter is a nutritional villain stands in contrast to research findings which have shown that it is the artificially hydrogenated vegetable oils in *margarine* which are implicated in both heart disease and cancer. A natural food that has been a component of many traditional diets for thousands of years, butter is a good source of fat-soluble vitamins A, D, and E, lecithin, and a number of important short- and medium-chain fatty acids.

Olive Oil. Olive oil, in which the fatty acids are largely monounsaturated and therefore chemically stable, is frequently recommended in the readings, to be taken in small amounts throughout the day or as a base for salad dressings. Unrefined, extra-virgin olive oil is noted as one of the healthiest oils for daily use; in fact, it has been credited in research studies with contributing to the low level of heart disease in Mediterranean countries, where olive oil consumption is high.

Gelatin. Gelatin is often recommended in the readings for its ability to promote the assimilation of nutrients from other foods. Powdered gelatin can be dissolved in a glass of water (drink before it jells) or stirred into salad dressings or sauces.[4]

Seasonings and Sweeteners

Seasonings are used sparingly in the Cayce diet, mainly in the form of sea salt or kelp, and cayenne rather than black pepper. Unrefined sea salt, available in health food stores, is a good source of iodine and other trace minerals not found in refined, bleached table salt, which often contains a number of undesirable additives. In contrast to black pepper, cayenne stimulates digestion without irritating the stomach. It facilitates the absorption of nutrients from foods and has a beneficial effect on the circulatory system.

Honey, raw and unpasteurized, is often referred to as the sweetener of choice in the Cayce readings. Along with easily digestible natural sugars, honey supplies small amounts of protein, vitamins, minerals, and enzymes. It also possesses antibacterial properties. According to Cayce, the intake of a small amount of honey may reduce excessive cravings for sweets in some individuals. Other options mentioned in the readings are beet sugar and brown cane sugar in moderation. Combining sweets with starches is not recommended.

Beverages

Water. The Cayce readings emphasize the importance of adequate water intake—between six to eight glasses each day. Water fulfills an important role as a nutritional catalyst. It is required for digestion and for the elimination of toxins and waste products. We depend on water to deliver nutrients to the cells and for the circulation of blood, lymph, and interstitial fluids. In several readings, the best type of water is specified as being mineral-rich mountain spring water.

Carbonated Drinks. In general, the readings advise against carbonated water and other carbonated beverages, the gases of which are said to be detrimental to the system. Most carbonated drinks today come in the form of soft drinks, which are loaded with refined sugars or artificial sweeteners of questionable safety. Cola drinks also contain caffeine, which, taken in excess, can overstimulate the nervous system and become habit forming. However, Coca-Cola syrup, taken in plain water in medicinal amounts, is considered helpful for purifying the kidneys and coordinating kidney and bladder action.[5]

Alcoholic Drinks. The Cayce readings advise moderation in the consumption of alcoholic beverages. Small amounts of wine, notably red wine, are recommended as a medicinal food, especially when combined with brown bread, preferably sourdough. In most cases, beer and other beverages brewed with hops are mentioned as being harmful, although one reading for a tuberculosis patient prescribes a daily drink made from beer and egg.

Coffee and Tea. The moderate consumption of coffee and tea is considered acceptable for most people, although coffee is said to have a higher food value. Note, however, that the readings are consistent in advising against the addition of milk or cream to either coffee or tea, since this increases their acidity. It is important to remember that caffeine, taken in excess, is an addictive stimulant that can wreak havoc with the nervous system. Furthermore, nonorganic coffee beans are often heavily sprayed with pesticides, which are not removed by roasting. Organically grown coffees, available in many health food stores, are chemical free and usually lower in caffeine. A number of flavorful coffee substitutes made from roasted grains or dandelion roots are also available. These are frequently mentioned in the readings as being preferable to coffee itself. Herbal teas are another good alternative for those who prefer to avoid caffeine.

The Multidimensional Dynamics of Eating

The importance of proper assimilation of foods is repeatedly stressed in the Cayce readings. Good nutrition is not just a question of *what* is eaten, but also *how efficiently the food is digested and utilized* by the body. The elements involved in this complex process include psychological as well as physical considerations. Essentially, they are all rooted in MINDFULNESS—in being fully present in the moment, conscious of the act of nourishing the body through eating.

Chewing and Taste. Probably the most important thing we can do to ensure that we assimilate the foods we eat is to chew our meals well. Chewing allows the starch-splitting enzymes contained in saliva to initiate the process of digestion. Chewing also increases the surface area of the food as it is broken down into smaller particles, making more of the food accessible to action by digestive juices. The better we chew our food, the less work the digestive system has in breaking it down further. Edgar Cayce suggested that even liquids should be chewed.

Chew any mouthful of food at least fourteen times. Even in drinking water, *chew* it—or masticate it at least three or four times. That is, sip it—let the activity of the glands in the mouth mingle well with the water; not gulping it but sipping it gently. 595-1

Chewing food well also allows us to become more aware of its taste. The experience of taste appears to be an important factor in maximizing the nutrition we derive from food. Marc David, in his book *Nourishing Wisdom*, tells of a research study in which scientists determined that absolute taste deprivation results in clinical malnutrition, even when nutritious foods are eaten. The researchers concluded that there must be important yet unknown physiological connections between taste and health. It is also interesting to note that the millennia-old Indian medical system of Ayurveda maintains that different taste sensations directly influence physiological function. Ayurvedic therapy involves a diet based on foods grouped according to taste in order to counteract energy imbalances in the body.

We also know that tension, fear, and worry inhibit the secretion of digestive juices, which results in incomplete digestion and poor assimilation. It is best to eat in a relaxed, peaceful atmosphere. If we take the time to consciously chew, taste, and enjoy each meal, we will be better nourished. And we may be less likely to eat junk foods, an unhealthy craving for which can arise from a lack of feeling satisfied by the meals we gulp down without fully experiencing them.

Attitude. The Cayce readings often remind us of the importance of holding the right attitude—toward ourselves and others, toward specific challenges and circumstances. Similarly, a positive and constructive attitude toward diet helps us to derive maximum nourishment from the foods we eat. Through our consciousness, the readings say, we can actively influence how the nutrients are processed in the body:

> That thou eatest, *see* it *doing* that *thou* would *have* it do. Now there is often considered as to why do those of either the vegetable, mineral, or combination compounds, have different effects under different conditions? It is the *consciousness* of the *individual body!* Give one a dose of clear *water* with the impression that it will act as salts—how often will it act in that manner? 341-31

A lack of dogma is also evident in the Cayce philosophy on nutrition. Though it provides specific guidelines on food choices, the Cayce diet also encourages flexibility and a sense of tolerance. We are reminded to strive for an ideal in the way of diet, but we are not to become slaves to our own nutritional programs. One of the traps many of us fall into when we become aware of the relationship between diet and health is establishing for ourselves a set of dietary rules according to which we label foods as being either *good* or *bad*. Once a particular food has been assigned to the *bad* category, we might even become critical of ourselves and others for desiring or eating that food. The more zealous we are in our conviction that we have found the one right way of eating, the more limited we become in our understanding of food and our interaction with it. Cayce warns us against such an attitude:

> As we find, keep this as the rule—rather than studying the diet in such minutia that the body be-

comes one that can't eat this, or can't eat the other! or this would hurt, or that would hurt, or the other would hurt! Because such an attitude becomes as chronic as a disturbing diet! 1601-1

The late spiritual teacher Hilda Charlton, who was a vegetarian and was noted for her ability to combine spiritual wisdom with lighthearted humor, illustrated this principle by saying: "I don't eat eggs, but I am not afraid of them!" She chose not to include eggs in her diet out of a deep reverence for life and all things living, but she did not become upset or worried when she discovered that a food she had eaten contained eggs.

The challenge for us, then, is one of finding the right balance—of recognizing that diet, while important, should not be allowed to dominate our lives in dogmatic fashion. A biblical quote from reading 281-31 appropriately sums up the Cayce philosophy on this subject: *"So it becomes that as the Master gave, 'Ye shall not live by bread alone but by every word that proceedeth from the mouth of the Father.'"*

Now, let's look at each of the components of the Cayce diet in greater detail.

2

Building Immunity Through Alkalinity: The "80 Percent Solution"

Be mindful that the diet is such that it keeps . . . toward alkalinity for the body at all times; for this will not only prevent infectious forces but will aid in keeping the blood stream in such a manner as to aid in eliminations . . .   523-1

IN ITS INCESSANT battle against deadly viruses and life-threatening infectious diseases, modern medicine is continuously struggling to develop more powerful vaccines and antibiotic drugs. Although billions of dollars of research funds are being poured into this pursuit, countless people around the world die every year from a multitude of viral and bacterial infections. The idea that the body can be protected against infectious diseases through diet alone seems naive and almost preposterous.

Yet this is exactly what Edgar Cayce told a twenty-three-year-old woman who was unsure whether she should submit to vaccinations prior to traveling from New York to the United Kingdom in 1935. When asked if inoculations against contagious diseases would be necessary for her, Cayce said, *"So far as the body-physical condition is concerned, the adherence to the use of carrots, lettuce and celery every day at a meal or as a portion of the meal will insure against any contagious infectious forces with which the body may be in contact."* (480-19)

The young lady who posed the question apparently felt that Cayce's answer was too simplistic. She asked again: *"Can immunization against [the contagious diseases] be set up in any other manner than by inoculation?"* Cayce remained firm in what he had already advised her, clarifying his answer somewhat: *"As indicated, if an alkalinity is maintained in the system—especially with lettuce, carrots and celery, these in the blood supply will maintain such a condition as to immunize a person."*

A bold statement with far-reaching implications. Everyone knows that lettuce, carrots, and celery are healthy foods. Most doctors and nutrition experts would even agree that they may help prevent certain degenerative diseases. Carrots are known for their high content of beta carotene, which has been shown to have a protective effect against cancer. And lettuce and celery supply a number of important vitamins and minerals. But beyond that, what is so special about these vegetables that could *immunize* those who eat them regularly against *contagious diseases?* The answer to this question, even as Cayce says, is that all three are highly alkalizing in the body. And what exactly does this mean? We must look to biochemistry for the answer.

The pH Balance

All fluids, including body fluids, have a measurable degree of acidity or alkalinity, depending on their chemical composition. The scale used to measure these acid or alkaline levels is the pH (potential Hydrogen) scale, which runs from 0 to 14. Values below 7 represent increasing acidity. Values above 7 represent increasing alkalinity. A value of 7 is neutral.

Most body fluids must be kept slightly on the alkaline side for optimal metabolic function. Blood should be at or near a pH of 7.4. Maintaining this alkalinity is so essential for survival that the body mobilizes its special buffering system to neutralize excess acidity whenever the scale tips. A vital link in this complex buffering system is the body's *alkaline reserve*. The body draws on alkaline mineral elements to help restore alkalinity in the system. However, the minerals in the alkaline reserve must be replenished regularly through food.

This is why an alkaline-forming diet is most important. All foods, after being metabolized, leave either acid- or alkaline-forming mineral elements in the body. Alkalizing foods are those which supply predominantly alkaline-forming minerals such as calcium, sodium, magnesium, potassium, iron, and manganese. Acidifying foods, on the other hand, supply predominantly acid-forming minerals like copper, iodine, phosphorus, sulfur, and silicon.

Most fruits and vegetables are alkaline-forming, whereas meats, grains, and most fats and dairy products are acid-producing. In order to maintain an optimal level of health, we should derive 80 percent of our foods from the alkaline-forming category and restrict the acid-forming foods to 20 percent of total intake.

A quick assessment of the typical North American diet, which is based on animal proteins and relies heavily on refined grains, shows us that for most people this ratio is reversed. An overly acidic diet disturbs the body's biochemical balance and results in numerous health problems ranging from minor discomfort to major illness.

Excess acidity in the body interferes with cellular metabolism, decreases lymphatic function, and slows down energy production. Metabolic and digestive enzyme function is disrupted, impairing digestion and allowing toxins to accumulate. As a result, the body becomes less resistant to colds, infections, and chronic diseases.

Susceptibility to Colds

Some people seem to be walking magnets for colds, "catching" every cold and flu virus they come in contact with. Others manage to sail through the so-called cold season without so much as a sniffle. What is it that makes one person more susceptible to colds than another?

This question is as interesting today as it was in Cayce's time. When asked, *"What causes colds? Can you give me a formula or method of preventing them, or curing them?"* Cayce's response was clear and simple: *"Keep the body alkaline! Cold germs do not live in an alkaline system! They do breed in any acid or excess of acids of any character left in the system."* (1947-4)

Cayce repeatedly pointed out that maintaining proper alkalinity prevents cold viruses from taking hold in the body:

No allowing of the system to become overburdened with acids in the system; being mindful of the diets that have been indicated, that the system is kept more in the order of alkalinity in the body. For with the alkalinity rather in excess than in the minority, we would find cold and congestion will have no activity or effect on the body; for the germ cold does not live or subsist or take hold in an alkaline-reacting effluvium in the body. 576-2

One of the bodily systems affected by overacidity is the lymphatic system. This is the body's major waste removal mechanism, and it also constitutes an important part of the immune system. Lymph fluid flows along a network of lymphatic pathways resembling the circulatory system of the blood. In fact, the lymph vessels originate in the small lymph capillaries directly adjacent to the blood capillaries. The lymph acts as a scavenger in the system, picking up waste particles from the cells and ensuring that they are broken down and eliminated from the body. Viruses and bacteria are also filtered out and destroyed by the lymph. For lymph fluid to perform its function optimally, it must have an alkaline medium.

Excessive acidity slows down the flow of the lymph, creating a condition known as *lymphatic congestion.* This manifests as enlargement, inflammation, and hardening of the lymph nodes, lymphatic vessels, and organs (spleen, tonsils, and thymus gland). With increased lymphatic congestion, immune response is lowered significantly, providing colds and other viral and bacterial infections with an easy entrance into the body.

Maintaining the body's alkalinity through diet is, therefore, essential for optimal immune function and can indeed provide us with a certain degree of immunity to a multitude of viral and bacterial infections.

As Cayce suggested, a good way to achieve this is to *"eat right! that is, about a twenty percent acid to eighty percent alkaline foods."* (263-8) This can be done by choosing eight out of ten foods from the vegetable and fruit group, and complementing these with appropriate amounts of proteins, fats, and starches.

ACID- AND ALKALINE-FORMING FOODS CHART

ALKALINE-FORMING FRUITS†	ALKALINE-FORMING VEGETABLES	ACID-FORMING VEGETABLES	ALKALINE-FORMING MISCELLANEOUS
Apples Apricots Avocados Bananas Berries (all except Blueberries and Cranberries) Cantaloupes Cherries Citrus (Grapefruit, Lemons, Limes, Oranges, & Tangerines)* Dates Figs Grapes Guavas Melons Papaya Passion Fruit Peaches Pears Pineapples Pomegranates Tomatoes (fully vine-ripened) †fresh and dried (unsulfured) fruits *Do not combine with cereals except whole-wheat bread in small amounts.	Alfalfa & other Sprouts Artichokes (Globe and Jerusalem) Asparagus Bamboo Shoots Beans (Green, String, Wax, and Lima) Beets Bell Peppers Broccoli Brussels Sprouts Cabbage Carrots Cauliflower Celery Chard Chicory Collard Greens Corn, Sweet Cucumber Dandelion Eggplant Garlic Kale Kohlrabi Leeks Lettuce (all types) Mushrooms Mustard Greens Okra Onions Parsnips Peas Potatoes (with skins) Pumpkin Radishes Rhubarb* Rutabaga Sea Vegetables (Dulse, Kelp, Kombu, etc.) Spinach Squashes Watercress Yams, Sweet Potatoes *Some authorities maintain that rhubarb is acid forming.	**Beans (dried)*** **Lentils*** **Garbanzos (Chickpeas)*** *Alkaline forming when sprouted* ## ALKALINE-FORMING DAIRY Buttermilk (fresh) Milk (cow, goat, or human; raw, unpasteurized) Whey Yogurt (fresh) ## ACID-FORMING DAIRY Butter* Cream Cheese Cottage Cheese* Milk (pasteurized, homogenized, boiled, canned, dried) *Butter and soft cheeses from organic raw milk are neutral or slightly alkaline forming.* ## ALKALINE-FORMING NUTS Almonds Chestnuts* Coconut (fresh only) *Authorities are divided on whether chestnuts are alkalizing only when fresh, or only when roasted.* **(All other nuts are acid forming.)** ## ACID-FORMING FLESH FOODS All meats (beef, fowl, lamb, pork, venison, etc.) All fish (including shellfish) *(NOTE: Only beef juice, blood, and bone – e.g., bonemeal – are alkaline forming.)*	Agar-Agar Apple Cider Vinegar (raw, unpasteurized) Coffee (organic, black, taken with food)* Egg Yolks Fruit Juices (fresh, unpasturized) Gelatin (taken with vegetables or fruit) Glyco-Thymoline Herbal Teas Herbs (fresh and dried) and most Spices (nonirradiated) Honey (raw, unpasteurized) Mineral Water (noncarbonated) Miso (fermented soybean paste) Sea Salt (unrefined) *Limit consumption to one cup per day.* ## ACID-FORMING MISCELLANEOUS Alcoholic Drinks Drugs (most prescription and nonprescription) Egg Whites Gelatin (taken alone or with water only) Soft drinks Tea (black) Tobacco Vegetable Oils * (processed, refined) Vinegar (white, processed) *Castor Oil and Extra-Virgin Olive Oil, as well as some fresh, cold-pressed, unrefined vegetable and seed oils, are considered to be neutral or alkaline forming by some authorities.*

ACID-FORMING FRUITS

Blueberries
Cranberries
Plums
Prunes
Sulfured dried fruits

ALKALINE-FORMING GRAINS

Amaranth
Millet
Quinoa

(All other grains are acid forming.)
NOTE: Sprouting reduces the acid forming properties of grains. Some sprouted grains are likely to be alkaline forming.

© 1999 by Simone Gabbay and Francis Sporer

The chart shown on the previous page lists many of the most common acid- and alkaline-forming foods, sorted according to recent and widely agreed-upon nutrition research. Charts in other publications may disagree and list some foods in different categories. These discrepancies are sometimes due to different research criteria or to actual variations of mineral values in foods. It is important to bear in mind that the mineral content of fruits and vegetables is dependent on the presence of these minerals in the soil. The same food grown in different locations with different farming methods may show considerable variance in nutrient composition. Organic produce grown in naturally fertilized, mineral-rich soil without synthetic pesticides has a higher ratio of alkalizing minerals and other important nutrients.

Fruits that are harvested prematurely are not allowed to ripen naturally and are therefore unable to fully unfold their mineral sugar potential. Ripe, alkaline-forming fruits have a sweet taste and aroma. Unripe fruits, on the other hand, taste sour and are acid forming. Tomatoes, which are botanically classified as fruits, are often seen green and unripe on grocery store shelves. The generally accepted logic is that green tomatoes ripen with time and gradually turn red. But they will never be as juicy or taste as sweet as tomatoes that were allowed to ripen on the vine. Nor will they be alkalizing in the system.

Edgar Cayce frequently warned against eating tomatoes that are not vine-ripened.

> Of all the vegetables, tomatoes carry most of the vitamins in a well-balanced assimilative manner for the activities of the system. Yet if these are not cared for properly, they may become very destructive to a physical organism; that is, if they ripen after being pulled, or if there is the contamination with other influences. 584-5

The readings say that when tomatoes are eaten out of season, canned tomatoes are preferable, provided the canning was done without preservatives, notably sodium benzoate. Tomatoes and other produce chosen for canning are usually ripe and preserved within hours of harvesting.

In general, all handling and processing—including storage, shipping, cooking, canning, and freezing—reduces the alkaline-forming values of fruits and vegetables. Harvest-fresh and fully ripe produce is always preferable. When not available, then fruits or veggies naturally preserved or canned in their own juices without additives may be a viable alternative that still provides considerable alkaline-forming properties.[1]

Another reason for the differences in acid/alkaline food charts is that the results of tests which measure whether a particular food creates an acid or an alkaline condition in the body can easily be misinterpreted. Dr. Theodore A. Baroody, author of a highly informative book with the provocative title *Alkalize or Die*, explains why asparagus, a powerful acid reducer, was previously considered to be acid forming. Asparagus promotes rapid detoxification in the body, leaving acid residues in urine specimens immediately following digestion. These acids, however, are not derived from the mineral elements contained in asparagus, but are produced as a result of the cleansing effect of the alkalizing forces supplied by it.

Balance Is Key

Although maintaining an alkaline balance is extremely important, we should not go overboard in our efforts to alkalize. Cayce said that excessive alkalinity is worse than excessive acidity. The body requires a certain amount of high-quality protein and fat every day for cellular maintenance and metabolic function, so acid-forming foods must not be eliminated altogether. Protein is also a vital link in the body's ability to bind toxins, which is necessary for maintaining a healthy acid/alkaline balance.

Cleansing diets or fasts during which only fruits and vegetables or their juices are taken can be a good thing when followed for short periods of time or under professional supervision and for therapeutic purposes. A long-term maintenance diet, however, does require the balancing influence of proteins, fats, and starches.

There is also a certain connection between sufficient protein intake and the body's ability to produce hydrochloric acid, which is secreted by the stomach to initiate the digestion of protein and other nutrients. Hydrochloric acid does not disrupt the acid/alkaline balance of other body fluids, but rather promotes it by ensuring proper digestion. Thus, ultimately, certain proteins actually increase alkalinity, as Cayce mentioned:

> To be sure, ordinarily proteins are considered acid-reacting. But the *activities* of proteins in the system, when not taken with starch, bring the necessity of the [hydrochloric] activity in their digestive forces. So when proteins such as from fish, fowl or lamb are taken, their final reaction through the lower portions of the duodenum becomes nearer to a normal balance of alkalinity. For alkalinity begins with the glands themselves in the mouth. Then with the entrance to the stomach we have a combination of lacteals and hydrochlorics, dependent of course—upon the nature of the foods or *more* so the *combinations* of same. 920-8

Acid-Forming Food Combinations

Acidity arises not only from an excessive intake of acid-forming foods but also from improper food combinations. In one reading, Cayce explained how such a condition had come about:

> As we find, there is rather an acute condition of cold or congestion from an unbalancing in the alkalinity of the system. Not by the foods themselves; rather the manner of their combination. For, as indicated, there should not be taken starches and sweets at the same meal, or so much together (That's why that ice cream is so much better than pie, for a body!) 340-32

In the same reading, Cayce made an interesting distinction in the effect of starches grown below or above the ground: *"Meats or the like should not be taken with starches that grow above the ground . . . Hence potatoes or the peelings of same with meats are much preferable to eating bread with meats, see? Hence they may be combined more together."* There is, indeed, an important difference between starches grown above ground and those which grow below. Potatoes and other starchy tubers are more easily digested than whole grains and legumes, which contain enzyme inhibitors and phytates that interfere with mineral absorption. Only proper preparation techniques, such as soaking, sprouting, sour leavening, and thorough cooking can deactivate the enzyme inhibitors and neutralize the phytates. Refined grains are a poor alternative, since they have been stripped of important minerals, vitamin E, and the vitamin B complex, which plays an important role in the digestive process.

A combination that Cayce often warned against is taking citrus fruits, which are highly alkalizing alone and in combination with each other, at the same time as starches, such as with a breakfast cereal. Whole-wheat bread in small amounts was said to be the exception to this rule. People often seem confused when they hear that citrus fruits are alkaline forming. Aren't lemons, oranges, limes, and grapefruit acidic fruits? They are indeed, but once ingested, their organic acids stimulate the production of alkaline digestive enzymes and buffers in the pancreas and the liver. Citrus fruits also supply generous amounts of alkalizing minerals and are therefore ultimately alkaline forming in the body. In combination with starches, however, they have the opposite effect. In reading 189-6, Cayce said: "*Citrus fruits, to be sure, are* not *acid-producing; they are alkaline-producing, unless combined* with *starches at the same meal when these are taken in the system.*"

Psychological and Spiritual Influences

Conditions of stress or strain within the body must also be considered as an influence that combines with the effect of foods. Cayce gave a fascinating discourse on this subject:

. . . we would find that at times there are various conditions and various foods that produce, under the stress and strain of activity, a varied effect . . .

When the body is under stress or strain by being tired, overactive, and then would eat heavy foods—as cabbage boiled with meat—these would produce acidity; yet cabbage *without* the meats would produce an alkaline reaction *under* the same conditions! The same would be true if there were fried foods such as fried potatoes eaten, when there is a little cold or the body has gotten exceedingly cold or damp, these would produce (if fried) an acid, and become hard upon the system; while the same taken as mashed or as roasted with other foods would react differently. 1411-2

This reading strongly reinforces the concept of a mind-body connection, demonstrating how mental and emotional energies interact with the physical to bring about certain conditions in the body. When we are mentally or physically exhausted, stressed, or otherwise out of sorts, we must be much more careful about what we eat, as there is greater potential for increasing acidity through improper food choices.

Emotions such as anger, fear, or worry can of themselves produce an acid condition in the body. A reading sheds further light on this process:

In the present, the unbalanced condition in the physical of the alkalinity and acidity has caused, and does cause, congested areas in the functioning of the body. These as to their sources have in the main arisen from anger (physical) produced by the activities of environs about the body; thus causing the throwing into the lymph circulation those poisons which reacted upon the general physical body-relationships with the mental and spiritual activities of the body.

For the glands secrete according to impulse from the emotional system. 294-208

An alkaline-forming diet becomes even more important under such conditions. In addition, we can seek out situations, activities, and surroundings which help to restore a state of harmony in the body-mind. This might include spending more time outdoors and in nature; getting enough sleep and exercise, which both relax and energize; as well as praying and meditating on a regular basis.

In *Alkalize or Die,* Baroody says that "constant vigilance against inharmonious thoughts and feelings alkalizes and constructs a stronger, healthier body." He explains how the body's response to harmonious music and agreeable colors, and an individual's positive attitude toward career and daily work can move the body toward a state of alkalinity. Dr. Baroody calls prayer the alkaline-forming sacrament, suggesting that "alignment with the Holy Spirit is the most powerful and rapid way of achieving an alkaline-forming reaction in the body."

Alkalinity and Its Relationship to Calcium Metabolism

Calcium is the most abundant mineral in the body, and it plays a vital role in the maintenance of the acid/alkaline balance. An adequate presence of calcium in the blood is required to ensure that the serum pH level is maintained at the critical level of 7.4. When chronic overacidic conditions in the body cause a drop in blood calcium levels, hormones produced by the parathyroid gland stimulate a mechanism by which the necessary calcium elements are pulled from the bones. Unless blood levels of this mineral are once again raised through calcium assimilated from food, bone calcium is not replaced, and this causes bones to become increasingly soft and brittle. An alkaline-forming diet that provides plenty of calcium-rich green leafy vegetables and ensures the mineral's optimal utilization is both the best source and the best preserver of calcium in the body.   ·

Foods that are high in phosphorus, such as carbonated soft drinks and processed meats and cheeses, should be avoided. Their regular consumption interferes with calcium assimilation and disturbs the body's acid/alkaline balance.

Another important factor in the interplay of calcium

metabolism and alkalinity is sunlight, which is essential for the production of vitamin D in the body. Without sufficient vitamin D, calcium cannot be metabolized properly. According to Baroody, a minimum of 30 minutes of direct sunlight every day is required for the body to produce adequate hormonal levels and to assist in the acid/ alkaline balance. Depending on skin type and seasonal conditions, it is wise to follow Cayce's advice to avoid midday exposure to the sun, which can be damaging. Early morning or late afternoon are better times for sunbathing and other outdoor activities in direct sunlight, especially during the hot summer months.

Equally significant, yet not widely recognized, is that the optimal functioning of the body's endocrine system also depends on the absorption of sunlight (including ultraviolet) specifically through the eyes. The parathyroid gland, which regulates calcium metabolism, is an important player in this complex network of glands. Photobiologist John Ott and optometrist Jacob Liberman are two scientists who have done extensive research in this area. In Liberman's book *Light: Medicine of the Future*, he explains that the excessive wearing of sunglasses contributes to a wide range of health problems by blocking certain portions of the light spectrum from entering through the eyes. To ensure the optimal assimilation of calcium and other alkaline-forming minerals, the use of sunglasses and other UV-blocking lenses should be restricted as much as possible.

The Cayce readings acknowledge sunlight's role as an important cofactor in the proper utilization of nutrients in the body. In reading 142-5 Cayce suggested: *"Keep the body under the sunlight, either directly or artificially, as much as possible. This for the strengthening of the blood supply and for the activity of the chrysalis, or of the forces as will build calcium in the system. Do that."*

Many holistic health professionals today recommend

the use of special full-spectrum artificial lighting during the winter months, especially in northern latitudes where sunlight is restricted. Direct stimulation of the eyes with full-spectrum light, including ultraviolet, is an effective therapy for those suffering from seasonal affective disorder (SAD).

Self-Test for Alkalinity

How can we know whether our bodies are too acidic or are properly alkalized? Choice of diet is evidently the best indicator. If we follow an 80 percent alkaline-forming diet that is complemented by high-quality proteins, fats, and starches, our bodies are probably well balanced in alkalinity. As an aid in evaluating the body's pH, Cayce recommended occasional self-testing with a pH indicator known as *litmus paper.* Reading 462-6 suggests that it is *". . . well at times to test the body with litmus paper, both through the spittle and through the urine, that there may be—as indicated—kept the tendency of the* balance, *rather than an excess in either direction."*

Litmus paper indicates whether a medium is predominantly acid or alkaline. A similar material, pH testing paper, gives a more detailed reading. A strip of pH-testing paper, moistened with the saliva or urine to be tested, will change color according to the level of acidity, which is easily interpreted by a color scale on the package. In a healthy, properly balanced individual, saliva pH is 7.4 and urine pH is slightly acidic at 6.4. Any variation from this norm indicates an imbalance.[2]

Robert R. Barefoot and Dr. Carl J. Reich, coauthors of the book *The Calcium Factor: The Scientific Secret of Health and Youth,* are convinced that pH testing with litmus paper also " . . . represents the most consistent and most definitive physical sign of the ionic calcium deficiency syndrome." In other words, the test is a good indication of whether or not the body is calcium deficient. The authors recommend caution, however, in evaluating such tests, because " . . . the saliva can be influenced by some recently consumed food, thereby producing a false positive test." They suggest that the chance of getting a false reading can be minimized by waiting two hours after putting anything in the mouth before taking the test. They also say that a test showing acidic results should be repeated two hours later for confirmation.

Glyco-Thymoline

Glyco-Thymoline, marketed as "an alkaline cleansing solution," is frequently recommended in the Cayce readings as an alkalizing substance to reduce excess acidity in the body. The product is still commercially available today.[3] Although Glyco-Thymoline is primarily intended for use as a mouthwash and gargle, the readings suggest that a few drops of this liquid taken in a glass of water will function as an intestinal antiseptic and help to maintain proper alkalinity:

> Also we would use an alkalizer for the alimentary canal . . . each day take three or four drops of Glyco-Thymoline internally, in a little water. Take this for sufficient period until the *odor* [of Glyco-Thymoline] may be detected from the stool. This will purify the whole of the alimentary canal and create an alkaline reaction *through* the lower portion of the alimentary canal. 1807-3

The Cayce-recommended dosage of a few drops of Glyco-Thymoline a day should never be exceeded. Taken in such small amounts, it is highly beneficial. In larger quantities, it would be toxic.

A Note on Stomach Hyperacidity

One of the most common digestive complaints today is excessive stomach acid, sometimes referred to as "acid indigestion." This is not to be confused with the excess acidity of other body fluids, which is different but not necessarily unrelated. Countless sales of over-the-counter antacid remedies attest to how widespread stomach hyperacidity is. Since acidic conditions in the stomach are necessary for proper digestion, the term "acid indigestion" is contradictory.

Hyperacidity in the stomach is actually a secondary reaction resulting from the regurgitation of bile from the duodenum back into the stomach. This occurs when there is insufficient hydrochloric acid in the stomach in the first place, a condition which delays the stomach's emptying time. Bile—which is secreted by the liver and passed into the duodenum, where it aids in the emulsification and absorption of fats—is extremely irritating to the stomach lining. Since bile is also alkaline in nature, it provokes a reflex secretion of hydrochloric acid in the stomach, setting the stage for what is perceived as "hyperacidity."

Commercial antacid tablets are not the answer. Their repeated use will, in fact, cause depletion of important nutrients, such as calcium, folic acid, and vitamin D. It is far better to address the problem at its source by improving digestion in the stomach.

Maintaining a proper acid/alkaline balance in the diet is the first step. Chewing all foods thoroughly is another. Adequate water intake between meals is also essential. Refined, processed, and all fried foods must be avoided. It is also important to avoid food combining that interferes with digestion, such as eating concentrated proteins at the same time as concentrated carbohydrates, especially those grown above ground (see chapter 4).

Supplementation with a good digestive aid containing hydrochloric acid and digestive enzymes is often helpful.

Many people who have a low output of stomach hydrochloric acid might unknowingly suffer from *hiatal hernia*, a condition in which the stomach is forced upward through a weakened, stretched diaphragm, seriously impairing the body's ability to properly digest and assimilate food. Baroody, who also wrote *Hiatal Hernia Syndrome: Insidious Link to Major Illness*, says that most cases of hiatal hernia are directly traceable to stress response. Emotions such as anxiety, anger, and frustration create tension in the stomach—and in the solar plexus, where the body's second largest number of nerve interconnections are located. The resultant contraction of the stomach and spasm in the diaphragm ultimately produce the hiatal hernia.

This leads to pinching of the vagus nerve, which extends throughout the entire body and is largely responsible for controlling the production of hydrochloric acid. When the vagus nerve is pinched, hydrochloric acid secretion is curtailed, resulting in incomplete digestion of foods, thereby catapulting the body into a state of malnutrition.

Mainstream medicine considers hiatal hernia to be largely untreatable, except with symptom-suppressing drugs and, in extreme cases, dangerous surgery. But Baroody has had considerable success in treating this condition with a natural foods diet that is based on 80 percent alkaline-forming foods, along with high-quality nutritional supplements, regular chiropractic treatments, manual adjustments of the hiatal hernia, and appropriate exercises.

The adequate output of hydrochloric acid in the stomach is of utmost importance for the proper digestion of foods. Symptoms of a disturbance in this process should not be indiscriminately suppressed with antacids.

The Alkaline Solution

Making the shift to an 80 percent alkaline-forming diet is the single most important step we can take in our quest for nutritional healing. Those who make the choice to eat this way often report having more physical and mental energy, improved digestion and metabolism, healthier sleep patterns, and a more positive outlook and attitude toward life in general. In short, THEY FEEL BETTER AND ARE HEALTHIER.

Dr. John Pagano, who has achieved major break-throughs in the treatment of psoriasis through an alkaline diet and other natural therapies, says in his book *Healing Psoriasis—The Natural Alternative:*

> It is nothing less than amazing to see how quickly a patient responds, in a positive way, when the shift from acidity to alkalinity takes place. Joints become more flexible and less painful, colds and congestion, as well as some allergies, often clear up, and the skin takes on a healthier glow with many blemishes disappearing. Results are lasting if a patient does not revert back to his or her previous eating habits after being relieved of these conditions.

Edgar Cayce often used the phrase "consistent and persistent" in describing the commitment an individual would have to make if success was to be achieved with a particular therapy. Pagano's observation confirms that the degree of healing obtainable through a health-giving, alkaline-forming diet is in direct proportion to the depth of commitment which we bring to it.

3

The Healing Power of Enzymes
in Raw and Sprouted Foods

Plenty of raw vegetables are to be taken. At least one meal each
day should consist wholly of raw vegetables, or almost entirely.

1993-1

IN 1942, THE mother of a three-year-old girl requested
a reading for her daughter from Edgar Cayce, who clair-
voyantly determined that the little girl was bothered by
pinworms. The reading then suggested that it would be
possible to rid the body of these parasites with a simple
dietary measure—the increased consumption of raw
vegetables and fruits: *"These [pinworms] will be eliminated if there will be taken rather regularly some lettuce
and some of such natures of green raw vegetables; raw carrot, raw fruits."* (2015-10)

The sleeping Cayce had sufficient insight into the psyche of a three year old to anticipate that the little girl might not willingly submit to this dietary regimen, so he also provided the option of medication to be taken under a physician's care. But the concept of curing pinworms with raw foods is intriguing, particularly because it is not generally taught in mainstream pediatric medicine.

It is well understood, however, that pinworms and other parasites are more likely to thrive in an unhealthy intestinal environment. We also know that a diet which includes raw foods on a regular basis, especially chlorophyll-rich greens, promotes good digestion and intestinal integrity. So from the perspective of holistic health and nutritional healing, Cayce's raw-foods therapy makes good sense.

The curative powers of raw vegetables, fruits, and their juices derive not only from the abundant vitamins and minerals they contain, but also from the plant enzymes they supply. Enzymes are specialized proteins present in all living cells. They are organic catalysts necessary for every biochemical reaction in the body. Enzymes can be divided into three major categories according to their function: *metabolic* enzymes, *digestive* enzymes, and *plant* enzymes.

Metabolic enzymes, generally speaking, are the maintenance workers of the body. They play an important role in cellular repair and organ function. All physical and mental activities, including the process of thinking, involve enzyme activity.

Digestion, the complex process of breaking down and converting the foods we eat into simpler substances then used for tissue repair and various other metabolic functions, relies on enzymes every step of the way. Digestion begins in the mouth, where chewing ruptures the cell walls of the foods, and enzymes are activated.

The starch-splitting enzyme *ptyalin*, contained in saliva, breaks down the complex polysaccharides into simple sugars. This explains why a slice of bread, chewed well, quickly develops a sweet taste. After being chewed and swallowed, the food mass is acted upon by enzymes produced in the stomach, pancreas, and intestines. The majority of enzymes, however, are manufactured by the pancreas. Digestive enzymes are highly specialized in their function. The enzyme *amylase* breaks down carbohydrates, *protease* breaks down protein, *lipase* breaks down fat, and *cellulase* breaks down fiber. *Lactase* helps to digest lactose, the milk sugar found in dairy products. The release of these enzymes into the digestive system is regulated by a precise supply-on-demand process dependent on the types of foods that are eaten.

Plant enzymes occur naturally in all fresh and raw fruits and vegetables. They greatly facilitate the digestion and assimilation of nutrients in the body. When fresh and raw foods are taken into the mouth, the chewing action ruptures their cell walls and releases the plant enzymes, which immediately initiate digestion. Raw foods possess the exact amount and types of enzymes necessary for their digestion. Thus, enzymes taken into the body with raw foods greatly reduce the demand placed on the body to produce its own digestive enzymes. This assists the body in conserving energy for metabolic processes, resulting in better overall health and higher physical and mental energy levels.

The overconsumption of cooked and processed foods—which are devoid of enzymes—places an enormous strain on the pancreas to produce digestive enzymes. Enlargement of the pancreas and other pancreatic conditions are common complaints today. The eminent nutrition researcher Dr. Edward Howell says this is a direct result of pancreatic exhaustion from efforts to manufacture the abnormally high amount of enzymes required to digest excessive quantities of denatured, overcooked foods. In his popular book *Enzyme Nutrition*, he writes: "When there are no food enzymes in the food you eat to predigest it, your pancreas must enlarge to give out more internal enzymes to do the job."

When this condition remains uncorrected, digestive capacity becomes seriously impaired, and the body has no alternative but to "dump" incompletely digested food particles into the bloodstream. Unassimilated proteins often produce allergic reactions; and undigested fats promote cholesterol buildup in damaged arterial walls starved for nutrients that remain unavailable because of poor digestion. It becomes a vicious circle with serious and far-reaching effects on health and well-being.

In order to correct these and other degenerative conditions, we need to substantially increase our intake of fresh and raw foods. Cayce's advice is as valid today as ever: At least one meal each day, preferably the noon meal, should consist of a raw salad prepared with a variety of fresh vegetables, such as lettuce, celery, carrots, watercress, beets, cabbage, radishes, onions, spinach, and tomatoes. If an entirely raw meal cannot be arranged, then a side serving of raw foods should be taken with two meals each day.

Plenty of chlorophyll-rich greens should be included daily. Chlorophyll, the substance that gives plants their green color, helps to detoxify the body. It also has blood-building properties and promotes the activation of enzymes. Green vegetables are an excellent source of minerals, vitamins, and essential fatty acids. Lettuce of the deep-green leafy variety, such as romaine, escarole, curly endive, or leaf lettuce, is preferable to head lettuce like iceberg, which contains fewer vitamins and minerals. Adding fresh tomatoes is recommended due to their high content of such nutrients as vitamins A and C, but only when the tomatoes are vine ripened and in season. All salad ingredients may be sliced, shredded, or grated and then, if desired, made more palatable with small amounts of a natural mayonnaise or olive oil dressing to which a few drops of fresh lemon juice or wine vinegar have been added. In some readings, it was suggested that gelatin be dissolved in the dressing to enhance nutrient absorption.

The readings offer the option of occasionally substituting fruit for the vegetables in the raw salad. Ripe, fresh fruits provide generous amounts of vitamins and minerals, easily assimilable because of the plant enzymes they naturally contain. Some tropical fruits are particularly rich in enzymes. Pineapple, for instance, contains significant amounts of *bromelain;* and papaya is high in *papain.* Bromelain and papain are powerful proteolytic enzymes. Synthesized concentrates of both substances are available in supplement form to assist those individuals who wish to strengthen their digestive capacity.

Recent research has shown that bromelain also offers protection against travelers' diarrhea by temporarily inactivating receptors on the intestinal wall, thereby preventing E. coli from attaching. In addition, there is some indication that bromelain may interfere directly with the toxins released by E. coli. In light of this new research, Edgar Cayce's enzyme-rich raw-food therapy for pinworms seems more scientific than ever.

Enzyme Supplements

A growing number of holistic health professionals today recommend enzyme supplements for improving digestion and nutrient assimilation. Dr. Howell and other nutrition researchers suggest that anyone who eats a considerable amount of cooked food can benefit from taking supplements of plant enzymes with each meal to

assist in the proper breakdown of those foods and to reduce the strain on the body's own digestive organs.
Howell is convinced that food enzymes add years to life,
and he claims that "by eating foods with their enzymes
intact and by supplementing cooked foods with enzyme
capsules, we can stop abnormal and pathological aging
processes."

Most natural food stores today carry enzyme supplements. These range from single enzymes, such as amylase, to full-spectrum plant-enzyme capsules and complex
formulations combining plant enzymes with digestive
enzymes from animal sources. The pure plant-enzyme
formulations are preferred by vegetarians who avoid
animal products for ethical reasons.

Such supplements are convenient and helpful, especially when the body's own digestive ability is seriously
impaired. In the 1930s, very little was known about enzymes, yet Cayce was once again ahead of his time when,
in 1934, he prescribed an enzyme supplement in one of
his readings. A forty-three-year-old woman suffering
from anemia and uterine tumors was told that enzymes
would raise her blood supply and improve her chances
of successful therapy. In her written response, the
woman told Cayce: "...*my sister went or phoned dozens
of drug stores here in D.C., and the druggists had never
heard of enzymes.*" (264-39 Reports)

After Cayce clarified in a follow-up reading (264-40)
which pharmaceutical company made the product he
had recommended, one pharmacist was eventually able
to obtain it. The digestive enzyme formulation known as
Ventriculin had just come on the market. Cayce recommended it in several readings. Ventriculin is no longer
marketed today, but, as mentioned earlier, there are numerous other digestive enzyme supplements available.

Juicing

The Cayce readings also advocate the frequent use of freshly squeezed fruit and vegetable juices as part of a healthy diet. Citrus fruits and their juices are particularly rich in vitamin C and bioflavonoids. Bioflavonoids work synergistically with vitamin C to strengthen capillaries, to scavenge destructive free radicals in the body, and to support immune function. All fresh juices, of course, are powerful enzyme boosters.

In reading 2520-2 Cayce said: *"Thus, we would have quantities of citrus fruit juices, or citrus fruits, as a portion of the diet more than once a day."* In another reading recommending citrus fruits, he said: *"In most of the fruits, take the pulp* with *the juices themselves . . . "* (2448-1) This is an important point to bear in mind. The pulp in citrus fruits is especially rich in bioflavonoids; therefore, straining it out before drinking the juice means losing out on some of the best nutrition citrus fruits have to offer. Pulp straining could be termed "juice refining"— whenever we refine a food, we strip away most of its nutrients.

Fresh vegetable juices, too, have become popular in recent years. Trendy juice bars are springing up in many locations, offering their customers refreshing, energizing drinks that pack a powerful, nutritious punch. Enzyme-rich juices extracted from such veggies as carrots, beets, celery, and parsley make a delicious vitamin and mineral cocktail, and the nutrients in these juices are readily assimilated by the body.

The medicinal value of fresh vegetable juices is widely known today as well. This is also asserted in the Cayce readings, such as the one that recommends fresh carrot juice alongside a noon meal consisting of raw veggies: *"At such a meal take . . . at least an ounce of pure fresh carrot juice. This also will aid, and prevent toxic forces being reformed when the organs have been stimulated to activity, and will aid also in reducing the blood pressures in the system."* (1224-3) In another reading, Cayce prescribed carrot juice along with massage as a remedy for a kidney condition: *"At least once each day take an ounce of raw carrot juice. Use a juicer to extract the juice from fresh raw carrots."* (243-33)

The right equipment—a quality juicer—is indeed essential for the success of any juice therapy. The most popular juicers (and usually the least expensive) are those which work with centrifugal force to extract the juice. The main disadvantage of this method is that it accelerates oxidation and thus speeds up nutrient loss.

Press-type and masticating juicers are more expensive but generally yield a higher-quality juice with more of the nutrients intact. Juices should always be freshly pressed and consumed promptly, since oxygen interacts with enzymes contained in the juice to begin the process of fermentation and destruction of nutrients. Canned, bottled, or packaged juices are usually pasteurized to deactivate enzymes and thus extend shelf life. As such, bottled juices lack the very ingredient which gives fresh juices their health-promoting properties: *enzymes.*

The way in which we consume fresh juices also determines how well they are assimilated. Each mouthful should be sipped slowly and salivated thoroughly before swallowing. In his foreword to *An Edgar Cayce Encyclopedia of Foods for Health and Healing* (compiled by Brett Bolton), renowned Cayce physician William A. McGarey, M.D., says that even carrot juice can be consumed in excess. He cites the advice of Cayce, who said to take an ounce of carrot juice, not "this whole quantity at once, to be sure, but sip it—take fifteen to twenty minutes to take this amount; or it may be sipped in smaller quantities but often through the day."

McGarey asserts that this method of taking raw juice

is more effective than the common practice of gulping it down in large amounts in the hope that more will be better. He holds the opinion that *"carrot juice has been used to excess by literally thousands of people in this country of ours."* He continues: *"I have seen the color of carrot in the palms and faces of people using this juice as a therapy."* Such orange tinting of skin occurs when the body is unable, because of insufficient bile, fats, enzymes, or other nutrients, to convert excessive amounts of orange-colored carotenes into vitamin A.

Internationally acclaimed naturopathic physician Jan de Vries has also found that the medicinal use of fresh juice can be extremely effective in very small amounts. He has told audiences of the medicinal value of the juice of a raw potato, for example, which is rich in enzymes and highly alkalizing. He says that squeezing the juice from a freshly grated, unpeeled potato and drinking it first thing in the morning is a highly effective ulcer remedy. A miracle cure? No, just enzyme activity applied scientifically and intelligently.

Another popular home remedy, effective as a general health tonic, is to squeeze a few drops of fresh lemon juice into a glass of water and sip it frequently throughout the day. This helps to promote alkalinity and to stimulate the enzyme activity of the liver and pancreas.

Fresh vegetable juices to which parsley or watercress has been added help to purify the blood and strengthen the organs of elimination. Small amounts of red beets and beet greens combined with carrot juice help to stimulate the digestive system and benefit the liver, gallbladder, and kidneys.

A multiple sclerosis patient was told by Cayce to drink fresh vegetable juices daily:

> During these periods the diets should be of easily assimilated foods; with plenty of vegetable

juices, especially—and beets and carrots should be stressed. Preferably use a vegetable juicer. Spinach, and all forms of such leafy vegetables, celery, lettuce and the like, should be a part of the diet. About three ounces of such juices should be taken daily, whether it is at once or several times during each day, have at least that quantity. 2070-1

Including the fresh juices of raw fruits and vegetables in our diets is an excellent way to obtain the vitamins, minerals, and enzymes we need to achieve and maintain health and high energy.

Enzyme Inhibitors and the Benefits of Sprouting

Seeds, nuts, legumes, and grains all contain enzyme inhibitors to keep them from germinating prematurely. When a seed sitting on the ground absorbs moisture from rainfall and sinks into the soil, its enzyme inhibitors are deactivated, and the seed begins to germinate or sprout. Thus, enzyme inhibitors are beneficial and biologically important for the survival of each plant species. However, within the human digestive system, this benefit becomes a detriment. The enzyme inhibitors in seeds, nuts, legumes, and grains interfere with the proper breakdown of such foods when they are eaten.

Several methods, long used in traditional cultures worldwide, are effective in deactivating such enzyme inhibitors. The best known are soaking, sprouting, sour leavening (for grains), and thorough cooking. All legumes and whole grains are made more digestible by soaking them in tepid water for several hours and then cooking them adequately. Nuts are easier to digest after soaking and will not feel as heavy in the stomach when pretreated in this manner.

Alfalfa, sunflower, and pumpkin seeds, even legumes

and grains, lend themselves wonderfully to sprouting, which dramatically increases their nutrient value. Protein, vitamin, and mineral content is multiplied in sprouted seeds, and the elimination of enzyme inhibitors releases the enzymes, which then assist in digestion and assimilation. Many individuals who find that eating beans, lentils, nuts, and seeds causes bloating and other intestinal complaints are relieved to discover that they can readily digest the sprouted versions of these foods. Sprouting is also an excellent way to ensure that we have a steady, fresh supply of raw foods on hand. Sprouts add crunch, taste, and above all nutrition to salads and sandwiches, and they may be added to soups after cooking. With a little practice and minimal effort, we can grow sprouts at home in the kitchen or pantry. Many varieties of ready-to-serve sprouts are available in most natural food stores and supermarkets.

Ann Wigmore, M.D., known as the late "living foods doctor," provided many innovative ideas for the use of germinated foods. The raw and sprouted food creations described in her books include a seed and sprouts soup, a raw sprouts loaf, and sprouted sunflower cookies. A physician and educator, Wigmore believed firmly in the healing power of raw and sprouted foods. In her popular book *Recipes for Longer Life* she wrote: "Modern living, with its cooked food, overstimulation, and destructive living habits, has made of our bodies clogged sewage systems (literally)." She was convinced that healing could be achieved with a return to a more holistic way of living, "particularly if we eat living foods."

Until her death in a house fire in 1994 at the age of eighty-five, Ann Wigmore was herself a shining example of the health-promoting benefits of living foods. Her legacy continues to be taught and practiced at the Hippocrates Health Institute, which she founded, in Boston, Massachusetts.

Sprouted wheat berries and other sprouted grains form the basis of Essene bread, a popular health bread named after the ancient mystical brotherhood. Instructions for making this bread are given in *The Essene Gospel of Peace* and involve germinating the grain (by soaking) and then exposing it to sunlight so that the "angels of water, air, and sunshine" can "make the germ of life sprout in your wheat." The grain is then crushed, formed into loaves, and baked in the sun. Less traditional versions of Essene bread, commercially available in many natural food stores, are baked in ovens but nevertheless prepared along these guidelines. The grain in this moist, chewy bread is much better digested and assimilated than nonsprouted grain, and its nutrient content has been multiplied by the action of enzymes.

Cultured Dairy Products

Enzymes are found in all fresh, uncooked foods, including raw milk products and raw meat. Traditional diets around the world usually include a certain amount of raw foods or those that have been rendered more digestible through natural fermentation or autolysis. In our modern society, eating raw meat is not advisable due to the risk of contamination.

Raw milk and unpasteurized dairy products are mostly unavailable today for the same reason. The heat treatment used during pasteurization ensures that the potential risk of pathological bacteria present in raw milk is eliminated, but it does so at a cost. Pasteurization destroys enzymes, including the all-important enzyme lipase, which helps to digest the fats found in dairy products.

Raw milk and the butter and cheese derived from it contain ample amounts of lipase. If they were allowed to remain unpasteurized, they would not be implicated in causing a buildup of cholesterol in our arteries. Nutrition researcher Sally Fallon writes in her book *Nourishing Traditions:* "Lipase in raw milk helps the body digest and utilize butterfat, and some have speculated that the rise in heart disease in the West is due to the fact that pasteurization destroys enzymes." She further explains that these enzymes "help the body assimilate all body-building factors, including calcium . . . [which] is why those who drink pasteurized milk may suffer nevertheless from osteoporosis."

This question of pasteurization was already an issue in Cayce's day, as is evident from the following reading, in which Cayce suggested an alternative to raw milk—namely a dairy product cultured with lactic-acid bacteria (such as yogurt or buttermilk):

> Raw milk, to be sure, is better—but pasteurized milk needs to have that added that will make for a better activity with the gastric juices, under the disorders as have been existent in the system. Those like the Bulgarian forces, as make for the proper reaction of the bacilli that becomes active with the gastric juices.[1] 404-2

When raw, unpasteurized milk is allowed to stand at room temperature for a couple of days, it doesn't spoil. Quite to the contrary—it improves! Certain bacilli present in raw milk interact with airborne bacteria to initiate a fermentation process which sours the milk into a semisolid pudding with a delicious sweet-sour taste. Pasteurization eliminates these naturally occurring bacilli, so this process cannot be duplicated with the milk that is commercially available today. However, other cultured milk products, such as yogurt and buttermilk, offer a similarly pleasant taste and many health benefits.

Fermented raw milks have played an important role

in the diets of many indigenous cultures for thousands of years. In the absence of refrigeration, the spontaneous fermentation process made it possible for organic milk products to be preserved and stored for later consumption. Varieties include yogurt (which originated in the Balkan region of Eastern Europe, kefir (Caucasus), and leben (Middle East).

The nutritional and medicinal value of milks fermented by the action of lactic-acid bacteria was recognized by physicians in the Middle East hundreds of years ago. However, it was not until the early 1900s that Nobel prize winner Elie Metchnikoff began his scientific investigation on the subject, after becoming intrigued by the extraordinary sturdiness and longevity of the Bulgarian people, who, he noticed, consumed yogurt regularly. He focused his research at the Pasteur Institute on lactobacilli, concluding that their presence in large numbers in the human intestinal flora was a major factor in the successful prevention and treatment of disease.

Lactic-acid bacteria and their cousins, bifidobacteria, are natural residents in the human intestinal tract. They help maintain a healthy intestinal microflora, and they promote nutrient assimilation and a strong immune system. Research has shown that the synthesis of several nutrients, including B-complex vitamins and calcium, is enhanced by the action of these "friendly" bacteria. These bacteria also appear to be effective in reducing serum cholesterol levels, as well as the risk of bowel cancer.

Faulty diet, stress, and pharmaceutical drugs (particularly antibiotics) can seriously deplete levels of beneficial bacteria in the intestinal tract, thus making it possible for undesirable yeast organisms, such as *candida albicans,* to invade and thrive. Numerous health problems, such as chronic fatigue, multiple food allergies, and hyperactivity in children, have been linked to yeast overgrowth in the intestines.

The regular ingestion of lactic-acid and bifido-fermented milk products such as yogurt helps to recolonize the intestinal mucosa with beneficial bacteria. The sleeping Cayce was well aware of this:

Also we would add Yogurt in the diet as an active cleanser through the colon and intestinal system. This would be most beneficial, not only purifying the alimentary canal but adding the vital forces necessary to enable those portions of the system to function in the nearer normal manner. 1542-1

The protein, fat, and milk sugar in yogurt and other fermented milks are predigested, thus reducing the strain on the body to produce digestive enzymes. This frees up considerable energy—or "vital forces," as Cayce says—for metabolic processes. The benefits of fermented dairy products are thus twofold: They preserve the body's enzyme potential and support the recolonization of friendly bacteria in the intestinal tract.

Yogurt is the most popular dairy product fermented with lactic-acid bacteria. Commercial yogurt is produced from pasteurized, usually homogenized, milk to which the lactic-acid bacteria *streptococcus thermophilus* and *lactobacillus bulgaricus* have been added. Some health food store brands are made from nonhomogenized milk and also contain *lactobacillus acidophilus* and *bifidobacterium bifidum*. It's easy to make yogurt at home using a store-bought culture.

When circumstances or dietary preferences make it impractical to consume large quantities of yogurt or other cultured milk products, lactobacilli or bifidobacteria in supplement form, available in natural food stores, are more convenient to ensure adequate daily intake. In some cases, Cayce felt that such supplements would be helpful. A tuberculosis patient was told: *"Take into the system yogurt, one tablet, three times each day."* (5703-1)

Traditionally Fermented Vegetables

Lactic-acid fermented vegetables, such as unpasteurized sauerkraut, offer similar advantages. Raw sauerkraut is available in health food stores or may be made at home by mashing shredded raw cabbage to squeeze out the juice, mixing the pulp and juice with salt and water, then packing it all tightly in a Mason canning jar and allowing it to stand at room temperature for several days. The naturally present lactic-acid bacteria then initiate the fermentation process, which converts the sugars and starches in the cabbage into beneficial lactic acid.

Lactic acid does not promote excessive acidity in the body as does acetic acid in synthetic vinegar or alcohol used in other fermentation processes. Lactic acid does destroy putrefactive bacteria in the intestines. Dr. William Fischer, author of *How to Fight Cancer and Win*, considers lactic acid derived from natural fermentation to be "the ideal substance for detoxifying the intestines." He adds: "While regenerating bowel flora, it tones the whole body and all the organs." Fischer also sees lactic acid as an effective tool in the fight against cancer, calling it "a chemical repressor that fights cancer cells but is not at all harmful to healthy cells." Lactic-acid fermented foods are often part of the dietary therapy in alternative cancer clinics.

Another popular cultured food comes to us from Japan. Natural miso, a pastelike condiment produced from cultured and fermented soybeans, is known to have many health benefits. In addition to being a concentrated source of many nutrients, including protein, vitamins, minerals, and essential fatty acids, it also contains natural digestive enzymes and other microorganisms which aid in digestion. Miso is used in soups and sauces and as a condiment for grains. As such, it is usually consumed in small amounts, as are all fermented foods in traditional cultures.

Eating naturally cultured and fermented foods is a wonderful way of giving the digestive system a break from internal enzyme production, while also supplying the body with a rich source of nutrients in an easily assimilable form.

Enzymes in Clinical Therapy

Research conducted during the past decade has shown that taking mixed enzyme preparations, such as a combination of pancreatin, papain, lipase, amylase, trypsin, and bromelain, can promote healing and shorten recovery time following surgical procedures and sports injuries. Shorter hospital stays, reduced pain levels, and reduced swelling were observed in groups of patients taking these enzyme combinations. And their fractures healed faster. One study concluded that taking enzymes prior to sports competition can offer a certain degree of protection against tendon and muscle injuries. Researchers have also found that such problems as bursitis, tendosinovitis, and tennis elbow can be helped or prevented with enzyme therapy.

Potentially promising applications for clinical enzyme therapy include the treatment of cancer and other degenerative conditions. Dr. Edward Howell says that there is abundant laboratory proof that the enzyme chemistry of cancer patients is profoundly disturbed. In a 1995 article on Systemic Enzyme Therapy in the *Townsend Letter for Doctors*, Dr. Hector E. Solorzano del Rio writes: "Enzymes have the ability to reduce the thick fibrin layer [in tumors] which is abnormally fifteen times thicker than normal. By reducing this fibrin layer, the stickiness of the cancer cells is also diminished, and by this means we can prevent metastasis."

The application of enzymes in the area of nutrition and healing is only beginning to receive the attention it deserves. In the less than seventy years since 1930—when only eighty enzymes were recognized—the number of known enzymes has risen to several thousand. We still don't know all there is to know about enzymes. What we do know is that enzymes are the agents of life and that without enzymes life would not continue.

4

Preparing Healthy Meals the Cayce Way

> Then when the vegetables for the evening meal are cooked, cook them only in their own juices, their own salts retained in same. Do not take meats save lamb or fowl, and these never fried. The vegetables would be cooked preferably in Patapar paper, served in their own juices . . .   1224-2

SINCE CAYCE'S TIME, technology has changed many of the ways we cook our foods and prepare our meals. Our increasingly hectic lifestyles have created a demand for timesaving kitchen gadgets, and for prepared foods and "just-heat-and-serve" meals from our supermarkets. Freezer shelves filled with microwaveable frozen entrees line entire walls in grocery stores. Even health food stores have jumped on the bandwagon and now offer their own lines of organic prepared foods, ranging from home-style canned soups and stews to frozen pastas and exotic desserts.

Another option we resort to occasionally—assembling meals from packaged, canned, and frozen ingredients—has been given its own fancy name: *speed scratch cooking,* a dynamic-sounding term aimed at promoting a stylish image for canned and frozen vegetables and fruits.

This quest for convenience often causes us to overlook a number of important questions:

• How does all of this affect the nutrient value of the foods we consume?

• Are the ingredients that go into commercially prepared foods equal in quality to those we use to cook with at home?

• What materials are the pots and pans used in industrial kitchens made of?

• And how is this food cooked anyway: has it been boiled, fried, or microwaved before packaging?

Questions like these are concerns for the health-conscious consumer, since all processing of foods significantly affects nutritional quality.

We saw in the preceding chapter that raw foods hold the greatest nutritional potential and should be included in our diet every day. But cooked foods are an undeniable part of our culinary tradition and heritage. They may also have certain nutritional advantages of their own, as indicated by recent research demonstrating that *lycopene,* an important carotenoid in tomatoes that appears to protect against certain types of cancer, becomes more bioavailable when heated in cooking or in the canning process. One could speculate that this is one reason Cayce often said canned tomatoes are preferable to raw tomatoes that are not fully vine-ripened.

Sometimes the cooking process does make certain nutrients more accessible, and the Cayce readings acknowledge this. When a pregnant woman asked whether cooking destroyed the calcium in foods, Cayce answered: *"To be sure. At times, but if the cooking is done in Patapar paper, so that all the juices are saved with same, then these are just as well—and, as indicated—at times more preferable, for they are more easily assimilated, and especially so during pregnancy."* (457-9)

In the Cayce diet, the preferred methods of cooking are those which minimize the destruction of nutrients and maintain the natural state of each food as much as possible. Cayce frequently advised that vegetables and meats should be cooked "in their own juices." Conventional boiling of vegetables in water destroys water-soluble vitamins, especially vitamin C, and dissolves organic minerals, which are then often discarded with the cooking water. To preserve these important nutrients, Cayce recommended that vegetables be steamed or, better yet, cooked in Patapar vegetable parchment. Patapar paper is available in some health food stores and from the Cayce product retailers listed in the Resources section. If not on hand, the more popular type of cooking parchment found readily in supermarkets may be substituted, although it is not as strong and is less durable. Only Patapar paper, however, is guaranteed to be manufactured from pure vegetable fiber.

Cooking with Patapar Paper

Patapar paper is a tasteless, odorless vegetable parchment, which permits the cooking of foods while retaining all juices. Patapar is nontoxic and is so resilient that it can be rinsed and reused many times. Vegetables, fruit, and even meat may be cooked in Patapar. The foods to be cooked are washed, chopped, and placed on a dampened sheet of parchment. The corners of the paper are folded around the food and tied together with a natural cotton string. The pouch is then inserted into a pot filled with two to three inches of boiling water, covered, and simmered at a low-to-medium temperature. After cooking, the nutrient-rich juices that collect in the pouch may be served together with the meal, or drunk immediately as a powerful vitamin and mineral cocktail.

The juice should not be discarded, since it is in this liquid that many of the nutrients are dissolved during the heating process. The Cayce readings sometimes placed greater nutritional value on these cooking juices than on the foods from which they are extracted.

> Vegetable juices, vegetables cooked in their *own* salts and not in water proper—cooked rather in Patapar paper would be preferable. All of those that carry the salts, as the vegetable salts, such as beans, lentils, cabbage (especially red cabbage) and all natures—but cooked in their own juices, and the juices as much as or more than the vegetables *still* taken! 308-6

The parchment method is superior even to steaming, because it prevents oxidation by sealing out light and air to a significant extent. When vegetables are steamed, it is wise to limit air exposure by keeping the lid of the pot closed. The steaming water should be preserved (it may be frozen) for use in stews, soups, or sauces. Regardless of whether the parchment or the steaming method is used, veggies should only be cooked until they are tender-crisp, as overcooking results in loss of flavor and nutrients. According to Cayce, vegetables retain more of their nutrients when each type of vegetable is cooked separately. They also retain a more authentic flavor and appearance that way.

Using a Pressure Cooker

When Cayce was asked about the use of a steam pressure cooker, he responded positively, saying that this method preserves rather than destroys nutrients. Pressure cookers are consistently recommended by teachers of macrobiotics, a widely acknowledged method of nutritional healing based on the Oriental principles of yin and yang. The use of a pressure cooker is favored in macrobiotic cuisine, especially in preparing grains and legumes, because steam pressure reduces cooking time and, consequently, the rate of nutrient destruction.

The more traditional method of cooking grains, dried beans, peas, and lentils is to soak them for several hours to remove enzyme inhibitors and then boil them in appropriate amounts of water, which is absorbed during the cooking process. Whole grains and legumes are rich sources of nutrients, but they are difficult to digest unless properly prepared. Cayce emphasized this when recommending a well-cooked breakfast cereal of wheat or oats to some individuals, as he did in reading 1419-5, which says: *"Crushed or whole wheat well-cooked, that is very well if it is* well *cooked; this means cooking for three to four hours—cracked or crushed wheat . . . At another time use oatmeal, but the steel cut oats—not the rolled oats. The rolled oats make for too much acidity. The steel cut oats would be well."* Cayce consistently said that steel-cut oats were preferable to rolled oats, which have lost some of their nutrients in processing.

Baking and Broiling

For the preparation of fish and poultry or other meats, the Cayce readings favored baking, roasting, or broiling; and they advise against frying. Frying requires the use of a cooking fat, which is one reason this method is warned against, and cooking meats in their own juices, with no additional fats or oils, is recommended. The chemical structure of vegetable oils used for frying, especially those that are polyunsaturated, is adversely affected by cooking at high temperatures, which promote the formation of harmful trans-fatty acids and other toxic substances. The charring of meats, which usually occurs during frying (and barbecuing), results in carcinogens being formed. Baking or broiling is much less destructive, and meats thus prepared are easier to digest.

Meats may also be cooked in Patapar paper, which naturally preserves the nutritious juices.

Seasonings

The superior flavor of foods cooked in their own juice eliminates or minimizes the need for seasonings. If these are desired, they should be added after cooking to avoid vitamin and mineral loss. In reading 906-1, Cayce suggested that *"the cooking of condiments, even salt,* destroys much *of the vitamins of foods."* Sea salt or kelp salt are preferred over refined table salt, which lacks nutrients and contains several additives.

It is important to realize, however, that even sea salt is often refined. Unrefined sea salt, available in natural food stores, usually has a gray appearance. It has a coarse texture, and its naturally present moisture tends to make the grains lump together. This type of sea salt supplies valuable trace minerals along with a lower sodium chloride content. Kelp salt, often recommended by Cayce, is prepared from dried and powdered kelp, a sea vegetable which is an excellent source of easily assimilable iodine and numerous other trace minerals.

When the pungent taste of pepper is desired or called for in a recipe, the readings recommend to substitute cayenne for black pepper, which is an irritant to the digestive system. Cayenne, on the other hand, is a nonirritating digestive stimulant, which is also used medicinally.

Seasoning vegetables with some butter after cooking

is another option approved of in the Cayce readings. All fats should be consumed in moderation; and, ideally, no additional fats should be used in cooking either meat or vegetables, as this causes undue stress for the digestive system. Reading 844-1 recommends a dinner based on *"well cooked vegetables, but not vegetables cooked in or with grease; those cooked in their own juices, as in a steamer or in Patapar paper. These may be seasoned well with butter, but not seasoned with bacon or with cooking meats of any kind."*

Cooking Utensils

The quality of our cookware is as important as the quality of our foods. On several occasions, the readings advised against the use of aluminum ware in cooking. Aluminum in a cooking pot tends to oxidize and combine with the foods cooked in it, particularly if the foods, such as tomatoes, release certain acids during the cooking process. When Cayce was asked whether aluminum cooking vessels were a detriment to health, he answered: *"To some; and dependent upon what's cooked in 'em!"* (340-31) A fifty-two-year-old man, a piano teacher who suffered from poor assimilations, was told to *"not eat foods prepared in aluminum at all; for, from the natural conditions and the supercharges of acids, the body will be allergic to the effects from aluminum upon foods—especially tomatoes or greens of any character or kind."* (2423-1)

Excessive aluminum is poisonous for the body. Traces of this metal found in brain tissue have been linked to Alzheimer's disease. Aluminum pots, pans, and coffee makers have no place in the kitchen of a health-conscious cook. Even nonstick coated pots and utensils should be avoided, since they scratch easily, allowing the coating chemicals to seep into the food. Stainless steel pots, lead-free glass, and enamelware are much safer choices. Asked if stainless steel cookware was harmless, Cayce responded: *"This is best, except enamel."* (379-10)

Canned and Frozen Foods

Fresh foods are always the preferred choice, but when lack of time and need for convenience make compromise unavoidable, people occasionally resort to canned or frozen foods. Cayce was not totally opposed to canned foods, provided they had been canned in their own juices and without chemical preservatives, notably sodium benzoate.

A 1997 study conducted by the University of Illinois Department of Food Science and Human Nutrition concluded that canned fruits and vegetables are nutritionally comparable to their fresh and frozen counterparts. In fact, the study showed that certain vitamins and minerals are occasionally present in larger quantity in canned foods. A close-up look at the canning process, however, reveals that some of these nutrients may not come from the food itself, but from an additive. A case in point is calcium chloride, which is often added to tomatoes to keep the pieces firm. Similarly, canning companies sometimes add ascorbic acid (vitamin C) to canned and frozen fruit in order to maintain color, resulting in higher overall vitamin C content, even though some of this vitamin is lost in the heat processing prior to canning and in blanching prior to freezing. It must also be remembered that canned foods are exposed to extremely high temperatures during the canning process, which destroys all enzymes.

There are very few references to frozen foods in the Cayce readings. Those that do appear are generally not favorable. When asked whether the freezing process kills certain vitamins and how frozen vegetables and fruits compare to fresh, Cayce gave an objective response:

"This would necessitate making a special list. For, some are affected more than others. So far as fruits are concerned, these do not lose much of the vitamin content. Yet some of these are affected by the freezing. Vegetables— much of the vitamin of these is taken, unless there is the re-enforcement in same when these are either prepared for food or when frozen." (462-14)

Mainstream nutritionists usually consider frozen foods to be equivalent to fresh in nutrient value. But in the holistic community, there are some serious dissenters, such as the widely respected nutrition teacher and author Annemarie Colbin. In her popular book *Food and Healing*, she asks: "What happens to plant cells when the water in them freezes? We can only assume that, much like a water bottle forgotten in the freezer, the cells will burst." Colbin believes that this bursting of cells is the reason frozen untreated vegetables are mushy and limp when thawed, having been destroyed at the cellular level.

Microwave Ovens

Most people can barely recall what life was like before the microwave oven. The convenience of meals cooked in seconds was so passionately embraced by our time-driven society when this appliance became available that we naively pushed aside any concerns about the safety of the device or the nutritional value of foods cooked in it. Even health-conscious cooks, who go out of their way to ensure that their meals consist of only the best and purest ingredients, often defeat their own efforts by subjecting their organically grown foods to microwave radiation.

Research has proven that exposure to microwaves changes the molecular structure of food. The meal or snack that comes out of the microwave oven may look the same as it did when we put it in there; but on a molecular level, dramatic changes have occurred. One of the changes is the suppression of amino acid hydrolysis. Another is that the isomer form of the amino acid *proline* is changed from the right to the left, which is physiologically incompatible. Holistically oriented nutrition experts have long been concerned about the possible effects these changes might have on the health of those who eat such foods, but published research in this area has not been extensive. In 1989, however, Swiss researchers demonstrated that pathological changes occurred in test subjects following the consumption of microwaved foods. Test subjects scored an increase in leukocytes, an indication of serious stress in the body. At the same time, there was a decrease in lymphocyte count greater than the decrease typically associated with food poisoning. Total cholesterol levels increased, and blood iron was reduced.

The Swiss research team also tested samples of microwaved cow's milk, noting several significant changes in quality. Among these changes were increases in acidity and sedimentation, a change in the structure of fat molecules, a reduction of folic acid content, and an increase in nonprotein nitrogen.[1]

For several years now, pediatricians and manufacturers of infant formula have advised parents not to heat formula in the microwave oven. The risk of uneven heating is one of the reasons, but another relates to the structural changes of amino acids mentioned earlier. The fact that microwaving is not recommended for infant foods is cause for concern that it may not be a wise choice for older children, adolescents, and adults either.

Food Combining for Optimal Assimilation

Healthy eating is not only a question of choosing the

right foods, but also of combining them properly. Different types of foods require different gastric secretions for proper digestion. We can avoid putting excessive strain on the digestive system by staying away from poor food combinations that result in the release of gastric juices directly opposing each other.

In reading 416-9, Cayce says it is *"the combination of foods that makes for disturbance with most physical bodies . . . "* He goes on to explain that *"the activities of the gastric flow of the digestive system are the requirements of one reaction in the gastric flow for starch and another for proteins, or for the activities of the carbohydrates as combined with starches of this nature . . . "*

Avoid Combining Starches

Starches are complex carbohydrates found in such foods as bread, pasta, dried beans and peas, corn, rice, and potatoes. The Cayce readings often advise against combining several starches at the same meal. Combinations such as potatoes with rice, bread with pasta, or any of these together with a starchy vegetable such as corn, are therefore to be avoided or minimized. Cayce also stressed that each vegetable from the starchy pod variety (dried beans, peas, and lentils) is best balanced with one or two leafy vegetables.

Diets high in complex carbohydrates have become popular in recent years, but an increasing number of nutrition experts now concur with Cayce's advice to eat starches in moderation. Although starches supply the body with needed energy, they stress the digestive system when taken in large amounts. Cayce said that excess starches in the diet *"make for a hardening upon the activity of the glandular system as related to the glands of the body."* (1268-2) Dr. McGarey suggests that such changes in glandular activity affect not only the endocrine glands themselves, but also other tissues in the intestinal wall which are involved in the process of assimilation. In his *Physician's Reference Notebook*, McGarey explains that "overeating starches is a prime cause of obesity and might create an abnormality in the assimilatory cells of the intestinal tract."

Recent studies have also shown that women who eat large amounts of starchy foods in the form of bread, rice, and pasta have the highest rates of breast cancer.

Starchy foods are usually eaten in combination with other foods. One of the most common food combinations in the average diet is protein and starch. Examples are meat and potatoes, or cheese and bread. According to the readings, this type of combination is detrimental: *"In the matter of diet, we would be rather warned respecting too great a quantity of proteins as combined with starches at the same meals, you see."* (1158-1) Cayce's advice is supported by the recommendations of nutrition experts Dr. Bernard Jensen and the late Drs. William Howard Hay and Herbert M. Shelton, all well-known advocates of the theory that proteins and starches are incompatible in the stomach and should be eaten at separate meals. Their independent research findings on this subject are described in several books, including Jensen's *Vital Foods for Total Health* and the popular *Food Combining for Health* and *Fit for Life*, the latter two based on the work of Hay and Shelton, respectively.

Many people who adjust their diets to eat starches and proteins separately find that this important step clears up any digestive complaints and results in a stronger sense of well-being and vibrant health. Substituting other vegetables, such as broccoli, kale, chard, or Brussels sprouts for starchier foods, makes the meal easier to digest and assimilate. It may not even be necessary to ban starches from a protein-rich meal altogether—it might be enough just to reduce their quantity. Also, as mentioned in chapter 2, Cayce said it may be less stressful to combine meat with starches grown below the ground, such as potatoes, than with starches grown above ground, such as rice.

The readings often mention the words "quantity" and "excess" where food combinations are concerned. This confirms that it is not so much the specific substance that we need to be aware of, as the amount in which it is taken. Reading 1014-2 says: *"Not an excess of starches at the times quantities of sweets are taken."* Combining sweets with protein foods, such as meat or dairy, is preferable to eating sweets with starches. Cayce illustrates this further in reading 416-9: *"If sweets and meats are taken at the same meal, these are preferable to starches. Of course, small quantities of breads with sweets are all right, but do not have large quantities of same."* Reading 340-32 explains that since there is no starch in ice cream, *"ice cream is so much better than pie, for a body!"* The readings say that moderate amounts of ice cream, and especially fruit ices and sherbets, which are not dairy based, are generally preferred over starchy desserts. Custards and puddings, especially those containing a natural sweetener such as unpasteurized honey, beet sugar, or whole cane sugar, are other alternatives.

The readings repeatedly emphasize that acidic yet alkaline-reacting fruits and their juices, especially the citrus family, should never be combined with starches, such as cereals, except for whole-wheat bread in small amounts. " . . . do not combine *cereals with the citrus fruit juices at the same meal."* (1601-1) Rather, these were to be alternated as breakfast foods on different days.

Above and Below Ground

Another of Cayce's food-combining guidelines calls for balancing each vegetable grown below the ground with two or three above-ground vegetables. This rule of thumb seems to be uniquely "Caycean" and relates more to the intangible energies of these foods than to measurable chemical reactions. But a closer examination reveals that Cayce, once again, seemed concerned mostly about providing a balance for the starchy below-ground vegetables, such as potatoes and yams.

> ... a well-balanced vegetable diet, with three vegetables grown above the ground to one grown below; though such vegetables as turnips, parsnips, beets, carrots or radishes may be included among those grown *above* the ground—that may be used either raw *or* cooked as the regular vegetables. But either Irish or sweet potatoes, or rutabaga (turnips and rutabaga will be different for this body!) are those vegetables to be warned of. 677-2

No Milk in Coffee or Tea

According to Cayce, milk should not be added to coffee or tea. Moderate amounts of clear coffee were considered to have food value, but the addition of milk or cream to these was said to interfere with the digestive process. On the other hand, if milk or cream were consumed at the same meal, but not stirred into the coffee or tea, the reaction would be different.

> Coffee or tea should preferably be without milk or cream, for again we find that the combination of the acids—or the tannic forces, the chickory, or the properties there are the food values to the digestive forces—becomes disturbing, when combined outside of the body. However, if milk and coffee are taken at the same meal—but not combined before they are taken—the gastric juices flowing from even

the salivary glands in the mouth so taking these *change* the activity so that the food values of both are taken by the system, in the activity through the alimentary canal. 1073-1

Sam Graci, nutrition researcher and author of *The Power of Superfoods*, says that coffee, when taken black and following a meal, has an alkalizing effect on the body since caffeine is an alkaloid. "I am not promoting coffee drinking," he says, "but if you do occasionally drink coffee, have it black, nondecaffeinated, and only following a meal. If you drink coffee on an empty stomach, it is acidifying since it is a stimulant of serum chloride."

Principles of food combining, whether found in the Cayce readings or in other sources, are intended to be seen as helpful guidelines, not hard-and-fast rules. After listing some of these principles in reading 416-9, Cayce said: *"These are merely warnings."* Indeed, foods belonging to both the protein and carbohydrate groups are concentrated sources of nutrients from which the body will only derive maximum benefit if it is allowed to process them without too many foods with similar demands competing for attention in the digestive tract. How well an individual can handle incompatible food combinations depends on several factors, such as genetic constitution, physical and psychological well-being, even climatic conditions and time of day.

As we learn to rely on food combinations that support rather than hinder the digestive process, we will reap the benefits with a leaner, healthier body which intuitively desires nourishing foods in the right proportions. Cayce sums this up in reading 2454-1: *"Include all kinds of fruits and vegetables in the diet, these in combinations of course—that agree with the body."*
What agrees with one body may disagree with an-

other. Guidelines can help us to identify which food combinations we should avoid or minimize for optimal digestion and assimilation.

Dietary Fats: The Good and the Bad

A popular trend in foods today is toward reducing and eliminating fats. Consumers eagerly reach for groceries labeled "low-fat" or "fat-free," confident that they are choosing a healthier product for building a slimmer body. The underlying presumption is that all fats are bad and that any fat eaten will automatically pile up in unsightly deposits of body fat.

The process is considerably more complex, however. While some types of fats present serious health hazards, others are crucial to our survival. Dietary fat is a highly concentrated source of energy and plays an important role in metabolism and in protecting cellular health. The fat-soluble vitamins (A, D, E, and K) and the carotenoids depend on the presence of fats for their assimilation. Fats are also precursors of hormones and prostaglandins.

In mainstream nutrition and in the media, there is much finger-pointing in the direction of saturated fats as culprits in the current epidemic of cardiovascular disease, high cholesterol levels, and obesity. Polyunsaturated fats, found in vegetable oils, are being touted as the better choice for the health-conscious consumer. Refined vegetable oils, margarine, and vegetable shortenings have replaced butter and lard in commercial baked goods and packaged foods.

But while the 1900s have seen a gradual decline in the consumption of saturated fats, the rates of heart disease and cancer during the same period have risen. In 1995, 41.5 percent of all deaths in the United States were attributable to heart disease. Many independent nutrition researchers refuse to accept the assumption that saturated fats cause cardiovascular disease, referring instead to the statistical correlation between the increased consumption of refined vegetable oils and other refined foods, and the increased incidence of heart disease.

In contrast to saturated fats, the polyunsaturated vegetable oils are chemically highly unstable. The fat molecules in saturated fats are saturated with hydrogen atoms, which protects them against molecular changes and rancidity. Saturated fats are solid at room temperature. In polyunsaturated fats, there are empty spaces in the fat molecules which tend to attract foreign hydrogen molecules, thus rendering unsaturated fats more vulnerable to molecular damage and rancidity. Polyunsaturated fats are liquid at room temperature.

Polyunsaturated vegetable oils break down quickly upon exposure to air, light, and heat. The deterioration process, initiated during commercial oil extraction, produces damaging free radicals, which have been implicated as contributors to degenerative disease and premature aging. In addition, commercially processed vegetable oils are highly refined, bleached, and deodorized to improve the oils' appearance and to neutralize odor and taste.

Further damage is done when vegetable oils are artificially hardened by hydrogenation. Hydrogenated fats are found in margarines, vegetable shortenings, commercial baked goods, and processed foods and snacks. These are true junk foods, since they contain trans-fatty acids, which are chemically altered molecules that disrupt the function of enzymes and metabolic processes in the body. Medical research has shown that trans-fatty acids raise serum cholesterol levels and contribute to cardiovascular disease. In 1994, a study out of Harvard said that trans-fatty acids found in margarine could be responsible for 30,000 deaths due to heart disease in the

United States each year. Unfortunately, the myth that margarine is a heart-friendly health food lives on, since its producers and marketers naturally have no interest in dispelling it.

In an article in the November 1992 issue of *Health Naturally* magazine, entitled "Butter, the Healthier Choice," Dr. Zoltan P. Rona asks: "How dangerous can margarine be? One study by Malhotra, published as long ago as 1967 in the *American Journal of Clinical Nutrition*, compared two populations in India where the only difference in the diet was the type of fat consumed. The population that used margarine instead of butter had a heart disease rate that was **fifteen times greater** than that of the population that used butter. A follow-up study twenty years later reported the same statistics."

In a 1995 article in *Health Freedom News* magazine, entitled "Butter Is Better," nutrition researcher Sally Fallon and lipid chemistry expert Mary Enig, Ph.D., say that *"butter contains many nutrients that protect us from heart disease."* They disagree with widely voiced concerns about the cholesterol found in butter and other animal fats, pointing out that cholesterol is a potent antioxidant (protector against oxidation damage) *"that is flooded into the blood when we take in too many harmful free radicals—usually from damaged and rancid fats in margarine and highly processed vegetable oils."* Fallon and Enig refute the notion that butter causes weight gain, explaining that *"the short and medium chain fatty acids in butter are not stored in adipose tissue, but are used for quick energy."* The fatty tissue in the body consists mainly of the longer-chain fatty acids, which are derived from polyunsaturated oils and refined carbohydrates.

Cayce recommended the moderate use of butter, either as a spread on whole-wheat toast or as a seasoning dotted on cooked vegetables. In reading 1770-7, he told a woman, *"A little fat, here, needs to be taken; especially as from butterfat or dairy products."*

Although the readings acknowledge the need for certain fats in the diet, they also advocate moderation " ... *keep away from too much greases or too much of any foods cooked in quantities of grease—whether it be the fat of hog, sheep, beef or fowl! But rather use the lean portions and those that will make for body-building forces throughout. Fish and fowl are the preferable meats. No raw meat, and very little ever of hog meat. Only bacon. Do not use bacon or fats in cooking the vegetables, for this body; for these tend to add to distresses in those directions of this segregation and breaking of cellular forces throughout the system."* (303-11)

Olive Oil

One of the safest oils for culinary use is olive oil, often mentioned in the readings as the oil of choice for salad dressings. Chemically classified as monounsaturated, it is much less prone to deterioration than polyunsaturated oils. Only those olive oils labeled "virgin" or "extra virgin" are unrefined and mechanically extracted without the use of heat. In recent years, olive oil has been the focus of several research studies prompted by the low incidence of cardiovascular disease in southern Mediterranean regions, where olive oil is consumed in considerable quantities.

The Cayce readings recommend olive oil for medicinal uses also; for instance, after the three-day apple fast and after the application of abdominal castor-oil packs to assist in gallstone removal. Current research confirms that olive oil reduces the production of cholesterol gallstones and promotes bile secretion, thus improving fat digestion and toxin removal by the liver. Olive oil's good fame is supported by centuries of safe traditional use, a status which modern refined and denatured oils cannot claim.

Cold-Pressed, Unrefined Vegetable Oils

Commercially processed vegetable oil should be avoided, but not all vegetable oils are bad. Most natural food stores carry a selection of mechanically extracted, unrefined oils which are stored in opaque bottles in the refrigerator. In their cold-pressed, unrefined state, these vegetable oils are excellent sources of certain essential fatty acids (EFAs), which are often missing in the typical diet today. Essential fatty acids are those which cannot be manufactured by the body and must be obtained from food.

Physiologically, EFAs are involved in oxygen utilization, in hemoglobin production, and in the regulation of metabolism. EFA deficiencies are linked to a multitude of ailments, including heart and circulatory problems, neurological disorders, arthritislike conditions, PMS, and chronic atopic skin problems.

A whole-foods diet rich in whole grains, nuts, seeds, and green leafy vegetables naturally supplies EFAs in sufficient amounts. But many individuals who have subsisted on a refined-foods diet for many years may need extra help to replenish their EFA reserves. Among the best sources of EFAs are the oils from the seeds of flax, hemp, safflower, sunflower, and sesame. These can be used in salad dressings, added to foods after cooking, or taken therapeutically as a supplement. They should be kept refrigerated and must never be heated or used in cooking, baking, or frying.

Eicosapentaenoic acid (EPA), found in the oils of some ocean fish, notably salmon, tuna, and mackerel, is a fatty acid which provides health benefits similar to those of EFAs. Medical research has established a connection between fish consumption and a reduction in the incidence of heart disease. A study published in the *Journal of the American Medical Association* in January 1998 showed that men who ate fish just once a week had a 52 percent lower risk of sudden cardiac death than men who ate fish less than once a month. Many health professionals today recommend that fish be included in the diet two or three times a week. Along with fowl and lamb, fish is one of the preferred sources of animal protein in the Cayce readings.

This discussion of fats confirms once again that natural, unprocessed foods are best. Consuming moderate amounts of butter and virgin olive oil, avoiding refined and hydrogenated fats, and paying attention to adequate EFA intake are healthy choices for most people.

Locally Grown and Seasonal Foods

Today's shopper in a typical North American food store is accustomed to seeing a wide variety of fresh fruit and vegetables on display year-round. Even in the depth of winter, we are not surprised to find strawberries or tomatoes in the produce department, although we know that these would not be growing in our home gardens or neighboring farmlands at that time of year. But do the berries we bring home in January look, smell, and taste the same as those we buy from a local farmer in June or July? Hardly. Their dry, white flesh and lack of flavor betray the fact that they were picked long before they had a chance to ripen, so that they could be stored and transported over long distances without spoiling.

Advice from the Cayce readings reminds us that *"shipped vegetables are never very good"* (2-14) and that we should emphasize instead locally grown fruits and vegetables in our diet, since this helps to "acclimatize" the body and align its energies with those of our environment. This fascinating concept transcends the purely chemical aspects of nutrition; however, even from a scientific point of view, we would be wise to follow Cayce's advice, since the absence of sweetness and low juice content so typical of transported produce are also indicative of significantly reduced nutrient values.

During the winter season, it is not unusual for fruits or vegetables to have been in transport or storage for two weeks or longer before they reach our table. During that period, a considerable amount of nutrients have been lost. Sophisticated storage and refrigeration techniques can do much to preserve freshness, but they cannot do so indefinitely. Some vegetables and fruits are more susceptible to nutrient loss than others. Green beans, for instance, have been shown to lose over 50 percent of their vitamin C during the first three days after harvest, despite optimal refrigeration. Broccoli, on the other hand, maintains most of its vitamin C during that period and under the same conditions. Any evidence of wilting is an indication that nutrient destruction is well underway.

Edgar Cayce once made an interesting comment regarding this process:

> As it is so well advertised that coffee loses its value in fifteen to twenty to twenty-five days after being roasted, so do foods or vegetables lose their food value after being gathered—in the same proportion in hours as coffee would in days. 340-21

Benefits of Local Foods

When we build our meals around locally grown foods, we shorten the time between field and table, thus minimizing nutrient loss. Taking advantage of what the local market has to offer makes good sense not only with respect to our health, but also for economic and environmental reasons: By supporting local farmers and merchants, we reduce our own food costs while contributing to the economic health of our communities. We also lessen the environmental impact created when foods are shipped, trucked, or flown in from faraway places.

With local produce, the consumer enjoys a certain degree of influence over how the food is grown, since local farmers are more inclined to respond to customers' demands to reduce or eliminate chemicals and synthetic fertilizers. The farther away we go to buy our produce, the less we know about the processes it undergoes before it reaches our stores. A case in point is fruit imported from South America, which may have been sprayed with DDT. Although the use of this chemical is banned in North America, it is still being manufactured here for export. Ironically, much of it returns to us—unlabeled, of course—on imported fruit.

Eating with the Seasons

Locally grown foods are also seasonal foods, perfectly designed by nature to provide just the right kind of nourishment required to sustain us at specific times of the year. In the spring, fresh greens like dandelion and sorrel help cleanse the body of toxins accumulated during the winter. In the summer, plenty of fruits, berries, and salad veggies invite us to eat a lighter fare. In autumn, a colorful harvest of sturdier fruits and vegetables inspires the cook to create hearty soups and stews or to skillfully store and preserve a selection for the coming winter months. By gratefully accepting the food offerings of each season, we synchronize our bodies with the rhythms of nature, a process which can be seen as an extension of the "acclimatization" concept referred to by Cayce.

Emphasis on local and seasonal foods is not unique to the Cayce diet. Other traditional systems, notably Traditional Chinese Medicine (TCM) and Ayurveda, teach that, in order to maintain health, we must live in harmony with nature and balance our body energies according to seasons and local climate. To a large extent, this is accomplished through foods and herbs with certain seasonal qualities. The widely acknowledged macrobiotic diet also prescribes local and seasonal vegetables whenever possible.

Home gardening, of course, is the best way to ensure a continuous seasonal supply of fresh, local produce. With some skill and time investment, the home gardener with access to a root cellar can store vegetables such as cabbage, squash, carrots, and beets for use during the winter season. Supplemented daily with a variety of fresh homegrown sprouts, the vegetables and fruits that are stored or naturally preserved reduce dependence on transported foods while allowing the gardens to enjoy a well-deserved period of rest and rejuvenation.

Internal Seasons

Seasonal cycles are represented not only in the phases of the year, but also in the changes our bodies undergo on a continual basis. Our dietary needs change as we change; so in order to stay healthy, we need to adjust our food intake accordingly, both with regard to the amount and the types of food eaten. By harmonizing our energies with nature's rhythms, we become more sensitive to our own "internal seasons," thus allowing our intuition to direct us to the diet which is most appropriate at any given time. However, in order to develop and strengthen the intuitive process and ensure that we are not misguided by unhealthy cravings or desensitized taste buds, we must first become firmly rooted in health through the regular intake of wholesome foods. Making local and seasonal fruits and veggies an important part of our diet is one of the surest ways of achieving this goal.

Daily Meal Samplers from the Cayce Readings

Reading 757-3

Mornings—citrus fruit juices, or the pulp with citrus fruit, see? with brown toast, whole-wheat.

Or, if the citrus fruit is not taken there may be used the dry cereal—and do not use sugar on same, although the milk may be used—but preferably use that which is well balanced in the vitamin forces, or the pasteurized milk, or dry milk that is made for such usages. However, do not use citrus fruit juices and cereals at the same meal!

At this meal there may be also taken a cereal drink.

Noons—preferably a whole *green* vegetable diet, consisting of such as lettuce, celery, radishes, or any of those that make for the weight—as well as a balance of the diets that produce the *cleansing* effects throughout the system, see? Raw cabbage, or raw spinach, or raw foods—peas that have been cooked, but not wholly cooked, see? Mustard greens—*any* of these. And there may be used with these a French dressing or mayonnaise, to make them more palatable.

Evenings—vegetables *well*-cooked, but be sure that for each vegetable used that grows under the ground, there are *two* used that grow *above* the ground, either in leafy vegetables or the pod vegetables, see? Meats in moderation may be taken. When taken, preferably mutton, fowl, fish, or the like—see?

Reading 135-1

Mornings—Only the citrus fruit diet, *changed* of course, at times, to the hard cereals, whole-wheat, whole rice, or corn—as the case may be; but *do not combine* these with the citrus fruits, or have them taken at the same meal! Milk, Ovaltine, or cereal grain extract, may be used as a drink.

Noon—More of the vegetables that are *raw*. These may be made into salads with salad dressings, especially with as much of the olive oil as is palatable and that will be assimilated with the character of foods. This would include lettuce, turnips, cabbage, and all of those that may be used as such. Tomatoes, if they are *ripened on the vine;* otherwise, those that are canned *without* preservative—or especially benzoate of soda. (Do not use such as use that as preservative.) These may be used, especially the juices of same. Any that are palatable, that are raw.

In the evenings—flesh may be taken in moderation, but none that does not have the hoof divided and that does not chew the cud. In these, these should not be rendered in other than their *own* fat, and should *not* be in any grease other than their own—whether boiled, fried, or roasted. This will, of course, include breads also. Rye, whole wheat, or it may be mixed. At this meal light wines or malt extracts may be also taken as drinks.

Reading 304-27
Mornings—citrus fruit juices, or the pulp and citrus fruit; either grapefruit or—occasionally an orange, but grapefruit is the better for the body.

Tomato juices occasionally at the breakfast meal would be very well.

With these may be taken egg, and toast that is not buttered too heavily—dry toast, whole-wheat; with coffee. These will be found well. Occasionally there may be taken a little crisp bacon with the egg, which will be found to be beneficial.

Noon—a general vegetable diet; those vegetables either well-cooked or those that are raw, that would include a small quantity of lettuce, celery, spinach, or *any* of these—with carrots and tomatoes.

It would also be well at this meal that there be browned toast, or whole wheat bread, with coffee or tea; coffee is preferable for the body.

Evenings—a well balanced vegetable diet, of at least two vegetables above the ground to one below the ground. In this would be included cooked carrots, or cooked potatoes—provided these are not carrying quantities of grease; that is, they should be boiled, or mashed, or the like. Some white potatoes may be included, you see. The meats that would be taken at this meal only would include, preferably, lamb or fowl. Occasionally there may be taken beef, preferably broiled; liver, or such.

Reading 3823-2
Mornings—citrus fruit juices; orange juice and lemon juice combined, pineapple and pineapple juice, figs; or the dried figs stewed, or the cereals that have more of the whole-wheat with raisins in same—though do not use citrus fruit *and* cereal at the same meal. Whole-wheat bread or cracked-wheat bread toasted, with a little butter. Ovaltine or Sanka coffee or milk.

Noons—whole green vegetables are more preferable to heavier foods, especially at noontime; and these should be taken raw, in the form of a salad; such as celery, lettuce, onions, leeks, tomatoes, peppers, radish, carrots and the like—raw cabbage, especially the sprouts or the like. And oil or salad dressing may be used that will make it more palatable for the body; and this should be with calcium—rather sodium chloride, that is iodized and more preferable for the calciumizing or working with the conditions necessary for recuperative forces of the body. During those periods when there is little of the activity, so that there are not the normal eliminations, well that the vegetables or fruits that are the more laxative in form may be used as a portion of the meal; such as rhubarb, figs, pears—of course, these should be either fresh or those canned without any superficial or artificial preservative.

Evenings—a well-balanced vegetable diet. The meats that would be included would be fish or shellfish or lamb, and occasionally wild game or fowl. However, none of these should ever be fried. It would be especially well at the evening meal to have *red* cabbage, provided it is prepared in its *own* [juice]—as cooked in Patapar paper, so that all the juices and vitamins may be retained in same. It should be the same with fresh beans, peas, lentils or beans may be a part of the diet.

Reading 462-6
Mornings—citrus fruits or cereals, with whole-wheat or brown bread.

Noons (or one meal each day)—raw, fresh vegetables.

Evenings—well-cooked vegetables, with a little meat occasionally; but all of these should preferably be prepared in their *own* juices, to make for better assimilation.

5

Food as Medicine

Be mindful that the foods are those of body and blood building. Beef juices would be well to be taken *as* medicine, not as a drink or as soup or food, but medicine; thus sipped—a teaspoonful once or twice a day—would be *most* helpful.   1736-5

DISILLUSIONED WITH THE ineffectiveness and dangerous side effects of modern pharmaceutical drugs, many people today revert to nature and its medicine chest of herbs and medicinal foods. Our grandparents and great-grandparents were much more self-reliant than we are today in dealing with various ailments. Their simple home remedies were often as close as the kitchen cupboard or herb garden. Modern naturopathy, herbology, and homeopathy derive many of their most effective medicines from such traditional remedies.

The Cayce readings ascribe medicinal value to a number of foods, sometimes suggesting unorthodox and quite unusual food-based remedies, such as a solution of used coffee grounds for massaging tired feet, and apple brandy inhaled from a charred oak keg for the treatment of tuberculosis and pleurisy.

In this chapter, we'll take a closer look at some of the most important medicinal foods mentioned in the Cayce readings.

Almonds

Among its cousins in the family of nuts and seeds, the almond has long held a kind of royal status. In the Mediterranean region, where almonds are cultivated, it is said that "no one who can fill his pockets with almonds need starve on a journey." Although probably referring to the almonds' trading value, this statement is true in another sense as well: The almond is a highly nutritious food. In addition to being an excellent source of dietary fiber, it supplies important amino acids and several minerals, notably calcium, magnesium, potassium, and phosphorus. The Cayce readings suggest that the almond *"carries more phosphorus* and *iron in a combination easily assimilated than any other nut."* (1132-2)

Almonds are rich in monounsaturated oils, which are relatively stable and not prone to rancidity. This high oil content ensures maximum availability of the fat-soluble vitamin E, which is present in significant amounts. The powerful antioxidant properties of this vitamin further protect the oils from spoiling. The B-complex vitamins, as well as carotene, which is converted to vitamin A in the body, are also found in almonds. Current research confirming the immune boosting properties of each of these nutrients lend support to Cayce's bold assertion that *"those who would eat two or three almonds each day need never fear cancer."* (1158-31)

What could possibly be a simpler prescription for cancer prevention? Cayce reaffirms the anticarcinogenic effect of almonds in the following reading:

> ... especially almonds are good and if an almond is taken each day, and kept up, you'll never have accumulations of tumors or such conditions through the body. An almond a day is much more in accord with keeping the doctor away, especially certain types of doctors, than apples. For the apple was the fall, not almond—for the almond blossomed when everything else died. Remember this is life! 3180-3

Adding a couple of almonds to our diet every day is easy. Almonds taste sweet and delicious *au naturel,* but they can also be enjoyed in other ways. Slivered almonds add texture and crunch to cereals, salads, and vegetable dishes. Almond butter, prepared by grinding almonds into a creamy paste, is a delicious spread on whole-grain toast or crackers. For those who are allergic to peanuts, almond butter is a welcome alternative to peanut butter, for which it can be substituted in various recipes.

Finely ground almonds add a gourmet touch to cookies, cakes, and pastries, and since almonds are virtually starch free, they help to reduce the overall starch content of sweetened baked goods. As noted in the preceding chapter, Cayce advised against combining quantities of starches and sweets.

Almond milk is a great boon for lactose-intolerant individuals who have difficulty digesting cow's milk. Basic almond milk is prepared by mixing three parts water (preferably purified or distilled) with one part almonds in a blender. For a smoother texture, blanched almonds may be used; but fresh, whole almonds in their skins are more nutritious. The addition of a natural sweetener, such as honey or maple syrup, and some vanilla extract will round out the flavor. Blend well for two to three minutes until the liquid has a smooth consistency, then strain if desired. The result is a tasty, highly nutritious drink that stores well in the refrigerator for up to three days. It may also be substituted in any recipe that calls for cow's milk. Blending almond milk with fresh or frozen berries, or soft fruit such as peaches, results in a wholesome alternative to a dairy milkshake. For those on a tight schedule, commercially prepared almond milk in a variety of flavors is available in many natural food stores.

In addition to its many applications as a health food, the almond is treasured worldwide as an effective natural skin-care agent. Pulp strained from homemade almond milk may be retained for use as a body scrub to remove dead skin cells and improve circulation. Alternatively, finely ground almonds may be combined with a little water and mixed into a paste to be used as a face mask.

Almond oil has a mildly sweet flavor, making it a suitable ingredient for baked treats or light salad dressings. Because it is predominantly monounsaturated, it stands up well to heat. Almond oil is also an excellent all-purpose skin and massage oil that may safely be used even on delicate baby skin. Almond cream, which has a base of almond oil, is recommended in some Cayce readings as a remedy for problem skin and sunburn.

Apples

The apple is a popular fruit. In 1997, the average American consumed a total of forty-six pounds of apples. Almost half the annual apple crop in the United States is processed into products such as juice, applesauce, and pie filling. Apples are a good source of vitamins A and C and also provide vitamins of the B complex. In addition, apples supply considerable amounts of calcium, potassium, phosphorus, magnesium, and fiber (including pectin, which has a gentle laxative effect). Most parents know that constipation in a baby or young child can usually be relieved quickly with a meal of applesauce.

Apples are also high in bioflavonoids, which are key antioxidant compounds produced by plant metabolism. A 1997 study conducted by researchers from Finland's National Public Health Institute, in Helsinki, concluded that flavonoids from apples, notably the flavonoid *quercetin,* played a critical role in decreasing the risk of lung cancer.

There are numerous references to apples in the Cayce readings. The surprising twist is that Cayce said that cooked apples are preferable to raw, except when raw apples are taken as part of a therapeutic three-day semifast referred to as *the Apple Diet.* (See below.)

Beware of raw apples, unless taken *only* as a diet for cleansing the system. Baked or cooked apples may be taken. 1048-4

Beware of apples, unless of the jenneting variety . . . 509-2

In *The Edgar Cayce Handbook for Health Through Drugless Therapy,* Dr. Harold J. Reilly explains that the "jenneting" variety "is an obsolete word that refers to those apples of a sheep-nosed nature such as Delicious, Oregon Reds, Arkansas Black, and Sheep Nose."

It is difficult to speculate why Cayce, with few exceptions, advised against eating raw apples as part of a general diet. One might hypothesize that because the raw apple has such a powerful cleansing effect on the body, it could interfere with the normal process of assimilation of nutrients from other foods. In the few cases in the readings where raw apples are recommended, it is emphasized that these should be tree ripened, and not eaten unripe. Baked or roasted apples are often recommended.

The Apple Diet was prescribed as part of the treatment for numerous conditions ranging from pinworms and epilepsy to overacidity in the body.

> . . . occasionally—not too often—take the periods for the cleansing of the system with the use of the *Apple Diet;* that is:
> At least for three days—two or three days—take *nothing* except *apples—raw apples!* Of course, coffee may be taken if so desired, but no other foods but the raw apples. And then after the last meal of apples on the third day, or upon retiring on that evening following the last meal of apples, drink half a cup of olive oil.
> This will tend to cleanse the system. 543-26

Another reading promised that the Apple Diet *"would remove fecal matter that hasn't been removed for some time"* (567-7), underscoring the powerful cleansing action of apples in the intestinal tract. Cayce said that one could eat as many apples as one wanted while on the Apple Diet. Drinking plenty of water is encouraged; even small amounts of coffee or a cereal drink are acceptable during the three-day fast.

Bob Revay, who experimented with the Apple Diet, summarized his experience in the November/December 1993 issue of *Venture Inward* magazine: "Completing the three-day apple diet delighted me. I felt better than I had in years. My eyes (which had always been a little bloodshot) were clear, and I felt lighter and more at ease physically." Revay reported that he ate an apple whenever he felt hungry, but that drinking water relieved some of the hunger. His biggest surprise, however, came about half an hour after drinking the recommended half-cup of olive oil on the evening of the third day. His skin began to look shiny and slippery, as though coated with olive oil. Revay discovered that the oil had migrated from the alimentary canal to all parts of his skin, suggesting that an intense cleansing had taken place throughout the entire pathway of assimilation.

In *The Edgar Cayce Handbook for Health Through Drugless Therapy,* Dr. Reilly says that he has found the cleansing routine of the Apple Diet to be the first step toward improving assimilation and elimination. When toxins are eliminated, the body has a much better chance of absorbing and assimilating nutrients from food.

When shopping for apples—for the Apple Diet or otherwise—it is best to look for those that are grown organically. Nonorganic commercial varieties are often sprayed with pesticides and/or coated with wax to preserve freshness. Washing does not remove the wax, which is why waxed apples should be peeled before eating.

Beef Juice

Beef and other types of red meat are known as "heavy" foods, which most people find difficult to digest. From a nutritional perspective, however, beef is a highly concentrated source of important nutrients, including iron, zinc, phosphorus, and the B-complex vitamins. Traditionally, beef has been described as having strengthening properties. The Cayce readings propose that one can benefit from beef's considerable nutritional potential without burdening the digestive system by drinking beef juice. Beef juice is not the same as beef broth, but is the actual juice from the meat extracted through the use of heat. Cayce suggested that beef juice could add *"the greater strengthening influence without the addition of weight or of heavy foods."* (1343-2)

Beef juice, Cayce said, was to be taken as a medicinal food. A teaspoonful sipped slowly two or three times a day was said to be a powerful health drink.

> . . . there is more strength and body-building in one spoonful of beef juice than a pound of the raw meat or rare meat or cooked! and the system will build more from same if taken in that way and manner. 1259-2

> . . . a tablespoonful of the beef juice, made properly, carries the same quantity of nourishment that you would have in half a pound of beef! What would be a half a pound of beef at once in the body? Take, then, a teaspoonful at the time—this would be much better, and take it every few hours. 728-2

Cayce's detailed directions for making beef juice are explained in Dr. McGarey's *Physician's Reference Notebook:* "Take about one pound of round steak preferably. Cut off the fat, leaving the muscle and pieces of tendon. Cut this then into half-inch cubes, and put it into a glass jar without water in it. The jar should be covered but not tightly. Then put the jar into a pan with water in it, the water coming about one-half or three-fourths of the way toward the top of the jar. Put a cloth on the bottom of the jar to prevent the jar from cracking. Let the water then simmer for three to four hours. Then strain off the juice which has accumulated in the jar, and the remaining meat may be pressed somewhat to extract the remainder of the juice. The meat will be worthless. Place the juice in the refrigerator, but never keep it longer than three days. The quantity made, then, depends upon how much and how often the juice is taken. It should be taken two or three times a day, but not more than a tablespoon at the time—and this should be sipped very slowly, taking perhaps five or ten minutes to use the whole amount."

Dr. McGarey adds that the beef juice may be seasoned to suit personal taste. The readings suggest eating a cracker (whole-wheat or crisp rye) along with the beef juice to make it more palatable.

Every effort should be made to obtain organic beef, since the feed given commercial livestock contains many additives, and the animals themselves are commonly treated with antibiotics and hormones. Many natural food stores, specialty stores, and some supermarkets now offer natural alternatives.

Gelatin

The Cayce readings often recommend gelatin for its ability to promote the assimilation of nutrients from other foods. Cayce explained it like this: *"It isn't the vitamin content [of gelatin] but [its] ability to work with the activities of the glands, causing the glands to take from that absorbed or digested the vitamins that would not be active if there is not sufficient gelatin in the body."* (849-75)

Gelatin is derived from animal tissue, including bones and cartilage, that has been treated to produce pure collagen (a protein which is the chief constituent of the fibrils of connective tissue) in solution, and then evaporated to a highly concentrated gelatin liquor. The soft jelly that forms after evaporation is then dried, crushed, and blended. Gelatin is available in powdered form and in thinly pressed sheets.

Edgar Cayce suggested that gelatin should at times be taken together with raw foods and at other times on its own stirred into water. Reading 3405-1 says: *"In the diet include often those foods prepared with gelatin. Give gela-tin by itself also at least three times each week, at regular periods, about half a teaspoonful dissolved in water and taken."* A fifty-five-year-old woman who asked what she might do that would help her eyesight was told: *"If gela-tin will be taken with raw foods rather often (that is, pre-pare raw vegetables such as carrots often with same, but do not lose the juice from the carrots; grate them, eat them raw), we will help the vision."* (5148-1)

Powdered gelatin may be mixed together with chopped or grated raw vegetables, dissolved in a glass of water *(drink before it jells),* or stirred into salad dressings and sauces. It is important to bear in mind that boiling gela-tin reduces its jelling properties.

Cayce recommended gelatin as a nutritional aid to complement the treatment of numerous conditions, ranging from anemia and arthritis to multiple sclerosis and Parkinson's disease. Although the Cayce readings describe its function mainly as that of a catalyst for vita-mins and minerals from other foods, gelatin does have a certain nutritional value of its own. The amino acids *arginine* and *glycine,* as well as the minerals calcium, magnesium, phosphorus, and potassium, are contained in gelatin. Dr. Bernard Jensen, author of *Foods That Heal,* considers gelatin to be one of the best sources of cal-cium, pointing out that gelatin *"is actually 45 percent cal-cium."* Dr. Jensen suggests that *"Gelatin is what you have to use to build up your body when you get arthritis, rheu-matism, osteoporosis, and so forth."* From the informa-tion contained in the Cayce readings, we might also deduce that gelatin helps the body to absorb calcium, since the neck and soft ends of chicken bones are con-sistently said to be the most assimilable sources of cal-cium. These parts of the bone also contain substantial amounts of gelatin.

Gelatin-rich chicken soup, prepared with stock made

by simmering chicken bones, is an old home remedy often humorously referred to as "Jewish penicillin." In recent years, research has confirmed the benefits of chicken soup for the treatment of influenza and other infectious diseases. Bone cartilage, notably from sharks and cattle, is used in the alternative treatment of cancer. Hydrolyzed gelatin in capsules and in powdered form is sold in health food stores as a nutritional supplement. It is considered to be helpful in the natural treatment of osteoporosis and joint deterioration.

The many benefits of gelatin are only beginning to be understood by nutritional science. Current research appears to confirm Cayce's view of gelatin as a *"quick pick-up for energy, aiding the system—from the assimilation of this, with the chemical changes in the body—in creating those activities through the assimilating and glandular force for the energies that create corpuscle tissue in body."* (2737-1)

Grapes

As a medicinal food, grapes are valued by traditional societies all over the world for their curative powers. In France, where grapes are cultivated extensively, some people eat little more than grapes in those autumn days when the harvest season is at its peak. Combining tradition with convenience and instinctive knowledge of what is healthful, they make effective use of seasonal, nutritional medicine to cleanse their bodies of accumulated toxins in preparation for a change of seasons. If we all followed their wise example, we might at last be successful in eradicating the annual plague commonly known as the "cold and flu season."

The Cayce readings suggest that grapes and grape juice have a toning effect on metabolism and help to restore proper eliminations. A fifty-year-old woman who suffered from faulty eliminations was told:

> . . . have as much as the body can possibly as-
> similate of *grapes!* every character, or all that may
> be taken of the grapes, and grape *juice.* This will act
> as an aid in reducing those tendencies for gas.
> When using the juice, extract it from the fresh
> grapes or else use Welch's Grape Juice—but eat as
> much of the fresh grapes as possible to assimilate.
> 2140-1

The cleansing action is due to several factors: Whole,
fresh grapes are a source of dietary fiber, vitamin C, and
the mineral potassium (which helps to promote good
bowel action and assists in maintaining the body's acid/
alkaline balance). Some B vitamins, namely thiamin, ri-
boflavin, and B_6, are also found in grapes; and the red
and purple varieties also supply iron.

In addition, grapes contain a large percentage of water, which helps to detoxify and nourish the cells of the
body. According to Dr. Gabriel Cousins, author of *Spiritual Nutrition and the Rainbow Diet,* the water supplied
by sun-ripened fruit is superior in quality and nutritional value. The reason is that water in such fruit has
been "structured" by sunlight, resulting in a change of
its molecular configuration, and this gives it a higher
solubility for minerals than unstructured water has.
Structured water is better for the body because it helps
to improve the function of enzymes and promotes the
assimilation of nutrients into the cells. Ripe, juicy grapes
are a particularly good source of structured water.

Grapes are a popular fruit for cleansing diets and
monodiets. In his book *Skin Diseases,* internationally renowned naturopath Jan de Vries writes about the detoxifying properties of grapes: "An effective method to
quickly remove the toxins from the body is a period of

fasting on a grape diet, which means what it says, i.e., no other food than grapes should pass the lips." He suggests that this diet be followed for a maximum of four days.

Cayce would agree. In reading 1703-1, he recommended a similar regimen: *"Some days, for at least three or four days, eat only* grapes—*morning, noon and night*—grapes! *Not with the seed, to be sure, but preferably those of the purple variety; not the larger but those that are good and* not *those that have been shipped or kept too long."*

In some instances, Cayce suggested that *grape poultices* should be applied across the abdomen during the period that such a grape diet is followed.

> Or the body may, under the existent circumstances, go on an entire grape diet—see, *entire* grape diet, for at least three-day periods; then to the regular normal diet that has been indicated. Quantities of grapes! And should there appear any disturbance in the stomach and duodenum through those periods, make a poultice of the grape hull and pulp—between cloths—and apply over those areas; or over the abdomen and liver area, you see. Make this about an inch and a half thick—that large a quantity, you see, all over. Plenty of water, but just grapes for three days—quantities—all that the body may eat. 757-6

In reading 133-4, Cayce specified that the grapes for the poultices should be raw and quite thick: *"But the grape poultices should be made a little thicker. Let them be an inch and a half thick rather than half an inch or spread. You see, the heat from the body will cook the grapes. Don't cook them. Apply them raw. Only mash them . . . with the hulls, yes, but mashed."*

The Cayce readings also recommended diluted grape

juice (two parts juice to one part water) as a balancing tonic in cases of obesity. This was to be taken half an hour before each meal and again at bedtime until the desired weight loss had been achieved. A thirty-four-year-old woman who was concerned about keeping her weight down asked Cayce why she had been advised to take grape juice. He answered: *"To supply the sugars without gaining or making for greater weight."* The woman then wanted to know whether the grape juice really did have a direct effect on weight reduction. Cayce's response: *"If it hadn't, would it be given?"* (457-8)

In *Physician's Reference Notebook,* Dr. McGarey explains the mechanism by which a gradual weight reduction would come about if the diluted grape juice were taken consistently and persistently over a long period of time: "Apparently this has a function of giving a type of sugar to the body tissues which does not promote weight gain. It was suggested that when the body was satisfied with this type of sugar, then those cells and glands in the intestinal tract that tend to change most foods to sugar would not be called upon to function in this abnormal manner. Only the passage of time and the replacement of these abnormal cells with those built in a normal manner would finally rectify the situation."

In Europe, the juice of red grapes is a traditional remedy for children who suffer from anemia and certain other debilitating conditions. The naturally occurring vitamin C promotes the assimilation of iron from red grape juice.

The more sophisticated version of grape juice—wine—is recommended in several Cayce readings as a tonic. Most often mentioned is red wine, to be taken in small amounts and combined only with dark bread. Reading 1005-16 says: *"Red wine is helpful if taken as a food—not as a drink. So an ounce of this in the late afternoon with brown or sour bread, or the Ry-Krisp, or rye bread, or the pumpernickel or the like—and sipped with the bread, but chewing at the same time—will be helpful."* Some readings indicate that red wine taken in such a manner will add blood-building properties and thus help to correct anemia.

In recent years, scientific research has validated Cayce's classification of red wine as a health food. Specific antioxidant compounds identified in wine, notably red wine, have been linked to the prevention of heart disease and cancer. *Phenolic compounds,* as they are called, were found to have the potential for reducing the harmful oxidation of LDL (bad) cholesterol and for inhibiting platelet clotting, which can lead to heart attacks. High concentrations of phenolic compounds are found in grape skins, seeds, and stems, all of which are utilized in the process of making red wine. Red wine, therefore, is a particularly rich source of phenolic compounds. A study published in a 1997 issue of *Science* reported that the phenolic compound *resveratrol* has cancer-inhibiting properties; and a 1996 study conducted in Spain linked wine, along with fish and vegetables in the diet, to a reduced risk of death from heart disease.

The antioxidant properties of grapes and red wine are thought to be responsible for what has been termed "The French Paradox": Despite "high-risk" diets rich in saturated fats and sugars, the people of France enjoy the lowest rate of heart disease among the top eighteen industrialized countries. This factor has been linked to their liberal consumption of grapes and wine, notably red wine.

The seeds of red grapes are also the basis of an effective antioxidant supplement that has become popular in recent years. Grape seed extract, which contains high concentrations of a bioflavonoid complex known as *procyanidolic oligomers* (PCOs), is successfully employed in the treatment of arthritis, ulcers, arterial hardening, allergies, varicose veins, and numerous other conditions.

Honey

Throughout history, the nectar of the honey bee has been regarded as a nutritional delicacy and a medicinal food capable of healing the body and soothing the spirit. In Greek and Roman mythology, ambrosia—the food thought to confer immortality to the gods—is said to be honey or a mixture of honey and bee pollen. In the Bible, the "Promised Land" is also referred to as "the land that floweth with milk and honey."

Honey also has a long history as a component of folk remedies for various ailments, including colds, coughs, and other respiratory problems; digestive difficulties; and general weakness. East Indian Ayurvedic medical tradition values honey as a blood purifier, a decongestant, and a kidney tonic. The medicinal applications of honey were explored extensively by the ancient Egyptians. *Dian Dincin Buchman's Herbal Remedies* states that "no fewer than 500 out of 900 known Egyptian medical formulas are based on honey." Honey has also traditionally been used to dress wounds.

The Cayce readings consistently point to honey as the preferred sweetener, particularly when taken with the edible honeycomb. Honey was recommended to individuals suffering from a variety of ailments, including anemia, arthritis, diabetes, toxemia, and psoriasis. According to Cayce, honey has strengthening properties. The mother of an eleven-year-old boy, who requested advice for her son's diet, was told: *"Let the sweets be taken in such forms as of honey . . . [This] is body building, also [supplies] energies that are well for a growing, developing body."* (1188-11)

Cayce also indicated that honey may naturally suppress the desire for other sweets. An epileptic with an excessive craving for sweets was told: *"Once a day, early of morning, take a teaspoonful of honey (teaspoonful, not a tablespoonful), and there will not be the desire so much for other sweets."* (2153-4)

And a fifty-two-year-old woman suffering from insomnia was advised to take *"each evening before retiring, about a cupful of heated milk (raw milk, preferably), in which there would be stirred a level teaspoonful of pure honey."* The reading cautions: *"Do not boil the milk, but just let it come to the heating point, and then stir in the honey."* (2057-1) In folk medicine around the world, the combination of warm milk and honey is well known for its soothing, relaxing effects.

Honey's nutritional profile holds a few surprises for those who believe that it's just another type of sugar. Although natural sugars make up nearly 80 percent of its volume, honey also supplies small amounts of protein, vitamins, minerals, and enzymes. Honeyologist Joe M. Parkhill, a professor of agriculture and author of *The Wonderful World of Bee Pollen*, says that honey is the only food that provides all the substances necessary to sustain life, including water. Parkhill credits the enzymes in raw honey with activating a number of biochemical reactions within the body, notably those associated with digestion.

Of the two main monosaccharides (simple sugars) found in honey, *glucose* and *fructose,* glucose is absorbed quickly by the body and is the only sugar known to exist in its free state in the body during a fast. This is because glucose is required by the cells for energy and is the main source of fuel for the brain. Fructose is absorbed more slowly, but both glucose and fructose are easily assimilated and do not require the assistance of salivary, gastric, or intestinal secretions. Honey in small amounts is tolerated by most diabetics and hypoglycemics. In contrast, refined sugars, which are disaccharides, must be inverted and broken down into glucose and fructose.

The color, flavor, and nutritional qualities of honey vary, depending on the floral source of the bees' nectar. Darker-colored honey, such as that made from buckwheat, usually tastes stronger and has a higher mineral content than the popular lighter types, such as clover honey. In a reading for a diabetic Cayce suggested: *"As regarding the honey and honeycomb, as is seen, a portion of this is of that same cellular nature. Small quantities may be taken with impunity, yet the greater portion of same should be comb made from clover and buckwheat, rather than from flower or herb, see? That is, see that the honeycomb as used is from the apiary that has this annex to same for the care of the bee making same."* (953-21)

Especially remarkable about honey are its antibacterial properties. Bacteria cannot survive in honey, whereas common refined sugar offers an ideal breeding ground for bacteria. In recent years, there have been reports of Manuka honey, a special type produced in New Zealand, being effective against *H. pylori*, the bacteria said to cause stomach ulcers.

Recent research, reported in a 1998 issue of the *Journal of Apicultural Research*, also confirms that honey, notably the dark-colored variety, is a rich source of antioxidants effective in the fight against disease-causing free radicals.

Honey is also a wonderful skin nourisher. Its strong antibacterial action partially explains its effectiveness in promoting wound healing when applied externally. An article by apitherapist Ross Conrad in a 1993 issue of *Health Freedom News* magazine hailed honey as a dramatic burn healer. Conrad reported on a study with 50,000 burn patients in China's national burn center. This study documented the progress of patients with deep second-degree and superficial third-degree burns covering up to 94 percent of their bodies. Within months of treatment with a honey salve, these patients' skin had not only been healed but was also virtually unscarred in contrast to conventional burn treatment, which leaves the skin "rough, scarred, and marked with patches of excessive or reduced pigmentation."

The best way to enjoy honey is in its natural form: raw, unheated, and unpasteurized. The heat used in pasteurization destroys honey's valuable enzymes and vitamin C, and with it much of the goodness of raw honey. And, as Cayce repeatedly emphasized, the most natural form of honey is comb honey, honey that comes in the bees' wax comb. The chewy comb is edible, and makes a wholesome snack that quickly satisfies a craving for sweets.

Jerusalem Artichokes

A gnarled tuber that resembles a knotty potato, the Jerusalem artichoke has no relation to the more popular globe artichoke. The first part of its name, Jerusalem, is equally misleading, since the name "Jerusalem artichoke" is said to have its origin in the Italian word for sunflower, *girasole,* so named because the top part of the Jerusalem artichoke resembles a sunflower.

The Cayce readings recommend the Jerusalem artichoke as a medicinal food for numerous conditions, particularly diabetic tendencies, but also for anemia, toxemia, and other debilitative conditions.

Many nutrition experts today agree that the Jerusalem artichoke is a helpful food for those with blood sugar problems. *Inulin,* a soluble fiber found in Jerusalem artichokes, stabilizes blood glucose levels, thus helping to prevent both hyperglycemia (high blood sugar) and hypoglycemia (low blood sugar). One of the readings given for a diabetic suggests that the regular use of Jerusalem artichokes may reduce and even eliminate the need for insulin medication:

> Instead of using so much insulin; this can be gradually diminished and eventually eliminated entirely if there is used in the diet one Jerusalem artichoke every other day. This should be cooked only in Patapar paper, preserving the juices and mixing with the bulk of the artichoke, seasoning this to suit the taste. The taking of the insulin is habit forming. The artichoke is not habit forming . . . 4023-1

Another diabetic was told in no uncertain terms:

> *Do not* take injections of insulin. If more insulin is necessary than is obtained from eating the amount of artichoke indicated, then increase the number of days during the week of taking the artichoke, see? 1963-2

Jerusalem artichokes may be prepared and cooked just like a potato, or used as a vegetable in soups, stews, and casseroles. They may also be eaten raw in a salad, preferably grated. As in the following reading, Cayce sometimes suggested that raw and cooked Jerusalem artichokes should be alternated in the diet:

> At least four meals each week should include the Jerusalem artichoke in the diet. One time this should be cooked, the next time raw. When cooked, prepare as you would a boiled potato; not boiled too much, but sufficient that it crumbles—and keep the juices of same in same. Hence, cook in Patapar paper. 2007-1

Dehydrated Jerusalem artichokes in tablet form are a convenient alternative when the fresh variety cannot be located or when circumstances make it difficult to include this vegetable in the diet on a regular basis.

Note: Those currently on prescribed insulin should not discontinue or reduce the dosage of their medication without consulting a physician.

Mummy Food

Mummy food is the name given to a mixture of equal parts dates and figs, cooked with cornmeal and water to make a smooth consistency. This unique recipe had its origin in a dream that Cayce had involving an Egyptian mummy. An annotation by Brett Bolton in *An Edgar Cayce Encyclopedia of Foods for Health and Healing* explains how the recipe for mummy food was born: "In 1937 this recipe was given to Cayce in a dream, by a mummy who came to life and translated ancient Egyptian records for him. Later, in trance, the dream was questioned, and again the identical experience took place: the preparation for the food was given exactly as it had been given in the dream and was said to be a 'spiritual food.'"

Directions for the preparation of mummy food are given in reading 2050-1:

. . . a combination of figs and dates would be an excellent diet to be taken often. Prepare same in this manner:

1 cup black or Assyrian figs, chopped, cut or ground very fine;

1 cup dates, chopped very fine;

1/2 cup yellow cornmeal (*not* too finely ground).

Cook this combination in 2 or 3 cups of water

until the consistency of mush.

Another reading (1188-10) explained that *"it is well for this body, or growing bodies, or elderly individuals also, for strength building and for correcting the eliminations, to use this* [mummy food] *as a cereal, or a small quantity of this with the cereal, or it may be served with milk or cream."*
In yet another reading it was said that cornmeal with figs and dates prepared with goat's milk had been the basis of the foods of the Atlanteans and the Egyptians (5257-1).

Black figs or Syrian figs are the variety most often recommended for use in mummy food. The fig and the date each have some unusual concentrations of nutrients, notably calcium, magnesium, and iron in figs, and magnesium and the B vitamins in dates. Combined together, figs and dates have an ideal ratio of calcium to magnesium (2:1). From a nutritional perspective, this calcium-magnesium content, along with the B vitamins from dates, would make the mummy food combination a perfect food to soothe the nervous system and relax the body. Since a relaxed body and mind are a prerequisite for entering a meditative state and connecting with one's inner spirit, this, on the biochemical level at least, might explain in part why the readings referred to this mixture as a "spiritual food."

6

Vitamins and Minerals

The vitamin stimulation should be in the food values, rather than in the vitamin tablets themselves.   3602-1

As we find this body in the present, there only needs be added a well-balanced vitamin addition or supplement.   1505-8

To Take or Not to Take: Nutritional Supplements

IN RECENT YEARS, the health food industry in North America and other industrialized regions has registered a phenomenal growth. New health food stores have opened up at a record rate. However, some of these so-called health food stores offer very little food; instead, they specialize in nutritional supplements—capsules, tablets, or tonics—which are designed to fill in the gaps created by our nutritional shortcomings. While some experts claim that we cannot possibly be healthy without such supplements, others argue that they are a waste of money. Whom are we to believe?

The Cayce readings do not advocate the indiscriminate use of synthetic vitamins and minerals. Generally, Cayce suggested that it is preferable to obtain nutrients from food sources as part of a well-balanced diet. At times, however, he prescribed nutritional supplements, frequently to be taken at specific times and alternated with regular rest periods, so that the body would not become languid in its efforts to synthesize nutrients from food.

All such properties that add to the system are more efficacious if they are given for periods, left off for periods and begun again. For if the system comes to rely upon such influences wholly, it ceases to produce the vitamins even though the food values may be kept normally balanced.

And it's much better that these be produced in the body from the normal development than supplied mechanically; for nature is much better *yet* than science! 759-13

In several readings, it is mentioned that supplements should not be taken until the eliminative forces of the body are fully restored, since the supplements would only add to the existing trouble if this advice were not followed. A questioner who asked whether she should take vitamin tablets was told: *"These are well to be taken when there is not a tie-up in the eliminations. When eliminations are set up, take same. But if these are taken under the stress of the lack of functioning of the eliminating forces of the body, these produce more hindrances than helpfulness. They are as boosters—and if you boost a pain—do you relieve it, or get more pain?"* (307-21)

Readings such as these indicate the need for nutritional supplementation, especially for certain individuals, and in specific circumstances. Cayce's instructions for taking such supplements might be somewhat unorthodox, but, even in Cayce's day, they were miles ahead of the position generally favored by mainstream dietitians then and now: that all vitamins and minerals can be obtained through diet alone.

Today, our need for supplementation may be greater than ever. Aggressive modern farming methods have left most of our agricultural soil severely mineral deficient, initiating a chain of nutritional imbalances in commercial crops and in the animals and people who eat them. When minerals in proper ratios are not supplied in the diet, the production of enzymes in the body is inhibited, and vitamins are unable to function properly. Supplementation therefore becomes an important option.

The nutritional supplements mentioned in the readings are mostly food based and thus highly bioavailable. One of these is wheat germ oil, rich in vitamin E and unsaturated fatty acids. Wheat germ oil is highly nutritious, but rancidity can be a problem if the oil is not absolutely fresh and properly stored in the refrigerator. Cayce also recommended cod liver oil, an excellent source of vitamins A and D. Calcios, a bone-meal-based supplement of easily assimilable calcium and several other trace minerals, is still available today. Unfortunately, others, such as Adiron, Kaldak, and Calcidin,[1] are no longer commercially produced. However, driven by consumer demand and enlightened research showing that wholefood extracts are preferable to the fragmented approach of taking isolated synthetic nutrients, the health-food industry now offers various types of concentrated wholefood supplements.

The following is an overview of the most effective ways of supplementing the diet with concentrated sources of nutrients:

Sea Vegetables.   One of the healthiest ways to add extra vitamins and minerals to the diet is through edible seaweeds. An excellent source of concentrated, easily assimilable nutrients, sea vegetables contain between ten and twenty times the amount of minerals found in land vegetables. They are also rich in protein and several important vitamins, notably A, B, C, and E. Edible seaweeds play an important role in traditional Japanese cooking, and they are extolled for their healing properties in the macrobiotic diet.

Most natural food stores today offer a selection of dried sea vegetables and can often provide cooking instructions, as well as cookbooks featuring recipes for seaweed cuisine. Some seaweeds, such as kelp and dulse, are also available in powder, tablet, or liquid extract form. The Cayce readings frequently recommend iodine-rich kelp as a food seasoning to be used in place of regular table salt.

Green-Food Concentrates.   The importance of including a variety of green vegetables in the diet cannot be overemphasized. Almost daily we hear of yet another research study which confirms that an increased intake of greens lowers our risk of getting cancer, heart disease, and various other degenerative conditions. Edgar Cayce consistently recommended green leafy vegetables as part of a healthful nutritional program. In recent years, several types of green-food concentrates, in powder or tablet form, have appeared on the shelves of natural food stores. These are rich in chlorophyll, which acts as an effective detoxifying and anti-inflammatory agent. They also contain a wide range of naturally occurring amino acids, minerals, vitamins, and enzymes—which, due to their synergistic action, are readily assimilated by the body. Green-food concentrates are typically derived from plants such as alfalfa, barley, or wheat grass, or from fresh water algae such as spirulina and chlorella. Some products contain a combination of several or all of these "superfoods."

Bee Pollen and Royal Jelly. Bee pollen is the male germ cell of flowers, herbs, and tree blossoms, which, like honey, is collected by bees as their food. Bee pollen gained public interest after Dr. Nicolai Tsitsin's study, in 1945, identified a majority of beekeepers among the centenarians in the Russian Caucasus whom he was studying as part of his research for the Longevity Institute of the U.S.S.R. The beekeepers' longevity was attributed to the fact that they had been consuming bee pollen in raw, unprocessed honey as part of their diet on a daily basis.

A nutritional analysis of bee pollen shows that it is a complete survival food, possessing some 185 known ingredients, including all amino acids, vitamins, enzymes, hormones, and fatty acids necessary to sustain life. Bee pollen is especially popular with athletes, who use it to increase physical stamina and endurance. An excellent whole-food supplement, bee pollen can be taken by the spoonful on its own, or blended with yogurt, juices, or shakes to make an energizing health drink.

Royal jelly, a creamy, milky liquid, is a salivary secretion of bees that is synthesized during the digestion of bee pollen. It is fed to the queen bee during her larval and adult stages, bestowing longevity and enabling her to produce over 1,000 eggs per day. As a food supplement, royal jelly is valued for its high nutrient content, including high-quality proteins and B-complex vitamins—notably pantothenic acid, which is important for proper adrenal function. Therapeutically, royal jelly is used to treat a wide range of ailments, including arthritis, rheumatism, severe stress, and exhaustion.

Herbs from Nature's Pharmacy. Medicinal herbs are some of the best sources of concentrated nutrients and can help to correct vitamin and mineral deficiencies. In addition to single-herb extracts and tinctures, most natural food stores offer a variety of synergistically formulated herbal combinations aimed at correcting specific nutritional imbalances. Edgar Cayce also recommended several unique combinations of herbs for specific ailments and therapeutic purposes. These are described and explained in the book *An Edgar Cayce Home Medicine Guide*, and many are still commercially available.[2]

The Role of Specific Vitamins

In order to meet the challenge of designing an optimal diet, it is helpful to have a solid understanding of the different components that make up our foods, as well as some insight into how they interact with each other in the body. This knowledge then enables us to make full use of the therapeutic properties of foods and supplements, while not neglecting the important aspects of taste and enjoyment traditionally associated with a nourishing meal.

Less than a century ago, the existence of vitamins and their role in human nutrition were virtually unknown. Today, vitamin supplements have become so popular that an entire fast-growing industry has been built around them. An extensive body of research confirms that we need to ensure an adequate intake of vitamins for optimal health.

Vitamins are organic compounds essential for the proper functioning of the body. They are involved in a variety of tasks, including the regulation of metabolism and the transformation of energy. Although they are required in minute amounts, their deficiency over long periods of time can produce symptoms of varying severity, ranging from digestive difficulties to skin problems and nervous system disorders.

Chemically, vitamins are classified into two groups:

those that are fat soluble (vitamins A, D, E, and K) and those that are water soluble (vitamins B and C). While the fat-soluble vitamins are stored in the fatty tissue of the body whenever their intake exceeds the body's immediate requirements, the water-soluble ones, which are excreted in the urine, cannot be stored as readily and must be continually supplied in the diet. They are also easily destroyed during the cooking process, and special care must be taken in the preparation of fruits and vegetables to preserve these important nutrients (see chapter 4).

Edgar Cayce defined vitamins as *"the creative forces working with the body-energies for the renewing of the body!"* (3511-1) A holistic perspective recognizes the function of each individual vitamin within the complexity of an interdependent cooperative system of nutrients.

Vitamin A. Vitamin A regulates cell structure metabolism and growth. It is important for proper visual function, including night vision. Healthy skin depends on adequate supplies of vitamin A, as do the mucous membranes of the eyes, the mouth, and the gastrointestinal, respiratory, and urogenital tracts. Vitamin A in the body increases resistance to colds and other infectious diseases.

Good food sources of vitamin A are egg yolks and whole dairy products, liver, and fish liver oil. Carotenoids, the precursor form of vitamin A, are also found in yellow, orange, and dark-green vegetables, which are consistently recommended in the Cayce readings. With the interaction of fats and bile from the liver, these substances are converted to vitamin A in the body. Carotenoids are also effective scavengers of free radicals, the unstable molecules resulting from oxidation. Beta carotene, the most popular of the carotenoids, has been the subject of many studies proving its effectiveness in the prevention of degenerative health conditions.

Symptoms of vitamin A deficiency include poor night

vision, eye and/or skin irritations, delayed or stunted growth, and increased susceptibility to infections.

When choosing a supplement, it is advisable to look for a natural form, such as fish liver oil or vitamin A palmitate. Any reports of vitamin A toxicity usually come from studies undertaken with the synthetic form. Halibut or cod liver oil are frequently recommended in the Cayce readings. Supplementation with beta carotene and other carotenoids is a possible alternative for vegetarians who prefer to avoid fish liver oils, but the presence of whole, natural dietary fats is required to convert carotenoids to vitamin A.

Vitamin B Complex. The importance of an adequate intake of B vitamins is stressed in the Cayce readings. Although all members of the water-soluble B-vitamin family are most effective synchronistically, each has a distinct function of its own. The most important B-complex vitamins are:

> Thiamin (vitamin B_1)
> Riboflavin (vitamin B_2)
> Niacin (vitamin B_3)
> Pyridoxine (vitamin B_6)
> Pantothenic acid
> Biotin
> Folic acid
> Cobalamin (vitamin B_{12})
> Choline[3]
> Inositol[4]
> Para-aminobenzoic acid[5]

The B vitamins act as coenzymes in carbohydrate, fat, and protein metabolism. They are important for proper brain function and mental health. Toning and soothing to the nerves, they have become popular as antistress vitamins.

Varying amounts of the B-complex vitamins are found in whole grain products, green leafy vegetables, brewer's yeast, legumes, dairy products, and meats, especially liver. The regular ingestion of cultured dairy products, such as yogurt, kefir, or buttermilk, appears to promote the synthesis of certain B vitamins in the body, notably of folic acid. The B vitamin sources favored by Cayce were steel-cut oats, whole grains, and yellow colored vegetables and fruits.

> Q. Do I need vitamin B? If so, in what form and dosage?
> A. It is preferable that this vitamin be assimilated by the system from the natural sources, rather than in concentrated or tablet form, see? All bodies need vitamin B, and this body especially—because of its energies and its serious activities at times, even to the detriment of the body's physical abilities!
> All foods that are yellow in color carry excesses of vitamin B. Then, include in the diet such as: yellow corn meal, yellow squash, yellow peaches, oatmeal, corn and corn products—but especially those that have been supplied with that to balance same are well; as Kix, as steel cut oats, as the regular parched corn, as popcorn and all its products. These are the *better* manners to take vitamin B—unless some conditions have become acute—which they haven't here. 1158-26

The last sentence in the preceding quote indicates that, in certain situations, a supplement might be necessary. This is further explained in another reading:

> B_1 is a vitamin not stored in body, but it is necessary that there be the consumption of such each day . . . the B_1 activity is much better taken in foods

than in the segregated pellets or capsules. When it is impractical for obtaining the foods with sufficient quantities for the daily needs, very well to take B₁. But to overstress same may at times cause the reaction of the *very* stress that is attempting to be aided! 257-326

What this reading further suggests is that when a supplement of B vitamins does become necessary, it is better to take a low-potency formulation, rather than the currently popular mega-B supplements. This sentiment is shared by a number of holistic health professionals today, who feel that low-potency values closer to the vitamin supply provided by food are better assimilated by the body.

Symptoms of vitamin B deficiency include general and muscular weakness, metabolic and digestive difficulties, and nervousness. If a supplement is called for, it is always best to take the complete B complex, and, if necessary, add extra dosages of a specific B vitamin that appears to be markedly deficient. It should be mentioned, however, that some individuals have an increased metabolic requirement for certain B vitamins, and they will continue to display deficiency symptoms until their need for greater intake is met or until their ability to assimilate and synthesize these vitamins is restored.

Vitamin C.   Vitamin C has become popular as an effective weapon in the prevention and relief of the common cold. It is also known as a powerful detoxifying agent and plays a major role in the production of collagen, a substance vital to the formation of connective tissue in the body. Vitamin C supports iron absorption and is involved in amino acid metabolism and hormone synthesis. This complexity of vitamin C's role may be what Cayce referred to in reading 5613-1, when he said that vitamin C produced "stamina *and* vitality *in the nerve* *centers and plexus"* and that its deficiency would result in *"a depleted nerve supply, and* from *same an* incoordination *in the functioning of the* organs *of the body as related to the replenishing or* resuscitating *forces of the system . . . "*

Vitamin C is abundant in fresh fruit, particularly in citrus fruit and berries. Other sources are green leafy vegetables, peppers, and members of the cruciferous family of vegetables, including cabbage, broccoli, and cauliflower.

When vitamin C occurs in nature, it is usually accompanied by bioflavonoids, such as those found in the peel and pulp of citrus fruits. When taken in supplement form, the effectiveness of vitamin C, also referred to as ascorbic acid, appears to be increased when it is combined with bioflavonoids. Current research involving bioflavonoids confirms their powerful antioxidant properties and identifies them as effective allies with vitamin C in the fight against free radicals in the body.

Vitamin D.   Of vital importance in the body's calcium and phosphorus metabolism, fat-soluble Vitamin D is unique in that it is produced in the body through the interaction of the ultraviolet rays of the sun with certain chemicals in the fatty tissue under the skin. This is by far the most natural and effective form of this "sunshine" vitamin, as confirmed by Cayce:

> . . . especially that that carries the vitamins that make for the building of the proper amount of calcium and the like, or vitamin D in the system, which will be found to be included in those that are well balanced in the sunshine—and keep the body in the sunshine; not so that there is injury to the body, but sufficient that all of the respiratory system and the capillary circulation is affected by the rays of the sun. 299-2

A marked drop in calcium absorption has been observed among residents of northern latitudes during the winter months, when sunshine exposure is restricted. Our predominantly indoor lifestyles—and the use of fluorescent lighting fixtures, which emit an incomplete spectrum of light—further reduce vitamin D intake and thus calcium assimilation. A woman wanting to know what changes in civilization were the causes for vitamin D deficiency was told: *"The tendency to have less sunshine activity, or less activity in the sunshine, and the taking of more foods that are not close to nature."* (658-11)

Food sources of vitamin D are fish and fish liver oils, and eggs and dairy products.

Deficiency symptoms include muscle weakness, nervousness, and irritability. The most severe symptoms are rickets and osteomalacia, the softening of bones in children and adults, respectively. Fish liver oil is a good choice for a natural-source vitamin D supplement. Cod and halibut liver oils are frequently recommended in the Cayce readings.

Vitamin E.   The subject of many research studies, vitamin E is a fat-soluble vitamin that has repeatedly demonstrated its effectiveness as an antioxidant and agent in the prevention of heart and lung disease. Vitamin E promotes the utilization of oxygen in the tissues and assists in the assimilation of vitamins A, C, and D. It also ensures the integrity of red blood cells. According to Cayce, vitamin E *"will act with the regenerative forces of the system."* (4246-1) This concept fits well into today's scientific perception of vitamin E as a promoter of youthfulness and longevity.

The best food source of vitamin E is wheat germ oil, which is recommended as a supplement in the Cayce readings. As Cayce pointed out, however, it is extremely important to ensure freshness, since rancidity destroys vitamin E and produces other harmful substances in the oil. Vitamin E is also present in many other unrefined, cold-pressed vegetable oils, as well as in whole-grain products, green leafy vegetables, and eggs.

Although a vitamin E deficiency is often difficult to pinpoint, symptoms such as heart disease, gastrointestinal problems, and sterility might be indicative of an insufficient dietary intake. The best way to avoid becoming deficient in this vitamin is to adhere to a diet that is fresh, natural, and unrefined.

When a supplement is called for, the natural form of vitamin E (d-alpha tocopherol) is preferable because it is far more biologically active than synthetic vitamin E.

Vitamin K.   Vitamin K, a fat-soluble vitamin, plays an important role in blood clotting by regulating the plasma content of proteins required for blood coagulation. There is also evidence that vitamin K promotes bone mineralization in the body.

The best sources of vitamin K are the dark-green leafy vegetables, such as broccoli, kale, spinach, watercress, and parsley. It is also found in some tuberous vegetables, as well as in egg yolks, liver, dried beans, and lentils. An extremely rich source of vitamin K is the herb alfalfa, available in capsule or tablet form.

Although about half of the daily requirement of vitamin K is synthesized in the intestines, a subclinical deficiency might occur in those who have a low intake of dark-green leafy vegetables. A marginal deficiency often goes unnoticed, since it will not immediately affect blood clotting ability. By increasing our intake of the dark-green leafy vegetables, as Cayce consistently recommended, and supplementing with a green-food concentrate, we can ensure that this important nutrient is present in sufficient amounts.

The Role of Specific Minerals

Although their importance in human nutrition is undisputed, minerals have not been in the spotlight as much as the more popular vitamins. Yet, without an adequate mineral supply in the body, vitamins are unable to do their job, and other biochemical functions are compromised. Minerals in the body are essential components of the skeletal system and other body tissues. They also play a role in metabolic processes and in the function of enzyme systems. They are required for the regulation of body fluids and for proper nerve transmission and muscle contraction.

Life cannot continue without such basic minerals as calcium, phosphorus, and iron. Major deficiencies can result when trace minerals such as iodine or zinc are lacking. Even an imbalance of the proper ratios of minerals required for human nutrition can predispose the body to illness.

Modern high-tech farming methods have depleted our agricultural soils' minerals. Chemical fertilization with isolated, improperly balanced mineral compounds wreaks havoc with the soil and facilitates the short-term growth of mineral-deficient crops. The mineral requirements of plants differ from those of humans, which is the reason a plant may be deficient in a mineral essential for human nutrition, even though the plant itself appears healthy. While not synthetically treated, even organically grown vegetables and fruit are not automatically a good source of adequate minerals in ideal ratios. Only with properly balanced soil chemistry can healthy crops be ensured.

The importance of soil minerals in nutrition and health cannot be overestimated. Dr. Alexander Beddoe, author of *Nourishment Home Grown: How to Grow Real Nutritious Foods in Your Back Yard,* says: "The longer I work with soil chemistry, the more I know that our poorly mineralized food is robbing people of life. Healthy and high mineral energy soil can have more effect on the health of human beings than all the medical institutions that will ever exist."

In the Cayce diet, special emphasis is placed on keeping the body in a state of alkalinity, which enables it to better utilize the minerals supplied by food. The actual mineral content of fruits and vegetables, however, ultimately depends on where and how they are grown. Cayce acknowledged this in reading 255-3, where he said that oranges grown in Florida (in his time at least) contained more iron than those grown in California.

Naturally, the best method of ensuring a high mineral content in our food is to grow it ourselves. When we must rely on commercial produce to meet our needs, the best indicator of its nutritional quality is taste. Healthy, mineral-balanced fruits and vegetables are more flavorful and aromatic. Their naturally sweet taste is indicative of a high mineral sugar content.

In planning our diets, we need to pay special attention to the minerals discussed below:

Calcium. Adequate calcium intake is a major nutritional concern today, especially for postmenopausal women, who are at high risk for osteoporosis. But calcium, the most abundant mineral in the body, is important for everyone. We depend on calcium for the development and maintenance of strong bones and teeth, proper muscle action, heart health, and a smoothly functioning nervous system. Calcium also plays a role in maintaining the body's acid/alkaline balance, as well as in blood clotting and other biochemical processes.

Even when major symptoms like bone loss are absent, a calcium deficiency in the body can cause numerous other disturbances, including muscle pains and cramps, anxiety, sleep disorders, and hyperactivity. As long ago as 1950, Dr. Carl Reich, a pioneer in preventive medicine, determined that common complaints such as indigestion, headaches, arthritis, and asthma could also be traced to a lack of calcium.

Of equal importance to the adequate daily intake of calcium is the body's ability to assimilate it. The maintenance of a healthy acid/alkaline balance with a diet consisting of 80 percent alkaline-forming foods is most important. When this balance is disturbed through the excessive consumption of acid-forming proteins and starches, the body tries to compensate by drawing on its reserve of alkalizing substances, including calcium.

The Cayce diet's high ratio of calcium-rich greens and other alkalizing veggies and fruits not only ensures an adequate intake of calcium, but also its proper assimilation. Green vegetables have the added advantage of supplying magnesium, another significant factor in calcium utilization.

Vitamin D, synthesized from the interaction of sunlight with certain chemicals in fatty tissue under the skin, is a most important agent in calcium absorption. Especially for those living in northern latitudes, a natural vitamin D supplement, such as fish liver oil, is essential during the winter months when sunlight is limited and outdoor activities are restricted. Sunlight absorbed through the eyes benefits the endocrine system, including the parathyroid gland, which regulates calcium metabolism. Therefore, sunglasses, which inhibit this process, should be avoided whenever possible.

Regular exercise increases circulation to the tissues and facilitates calcium assimilation. Massage offers similar benefits. Both exercise and massage also promote relaxation, a most important factor in calcium metabolism. Stress, worry, and tension, on the other hand, cause excessive dumping of calcium into the intestines, sometimes resulting in more calcium being excreted than is taken in with diet. Daily meditation, which helps us cope better with all types of stress, may be more important than a calcium supplement.

Calcium absorption is also reduced when high-phosphorus foods, such as carbonated soft drinks and processed meats and cheeses, are consumed with frequency. Excessive caffeine and sugar consumption has a similar effect.

Insufficient production of hydrochloric acid in the stomach is another factor that can significantly disrupt calcium absorption. A common health problem usually traceable to stress but most often associated with aging, this condition is relieved by taking hydrochloric acid in supplement form. An acid environment in the stomach—essential for the breakdown of nutrients—does not disrupt the acid/alkaline balance of other body fluids.

Once a healthy calcium metabolism has been restored, the body will readily absorb and assimilate this mineral from calcium-rich foods. In addition to leafy greens, these include egg yolks, dried beans, almonds, sesame seeds, dairy products, and kelp and other sea vegetables. Along with orange juice, Cayce recommended carrots and turnips for added calcium intake. He also considered chicken bones to be an excellent dietary source of calcium, which is best accessed by thoroughly chewing the bones, especially neck bones and the soft ends of leg bones.

The calcium supplement most often recommended in the Cayce readings, notably for pregnant women, is Calcios, which is still available today. During Cayce's time, Calcios was made from pulverized chicken bones; but because of problems with the supply of raw materials, the product is now derived from cattle bone and marrow, which appears not to have reduced its effectiveness. The digestibility of Calcios is enhanced by the addition of hydrochloric acid and natural digestive enzymes. A thin layer of Calcios may be spread on a cracker and eaten as a food about three times a week.

Cayce also recommended small amounts of limewater, an aqueous preparation of calcium hydroxide, as an effective calcium supplement for babies and children.

There are many other types of calcium supplements on the market. The better brands are formulated for maximum bioavailability. However, the rate of absorption for most of these products is still relatively low. Professor C. Louis Kervran, who has done extensive research on the issue of mineral absorption, argues in his book *Biological Transmutations* that the body is unable to assimilate elemental calcium but instead manufactures it from magnesium, potassium, and silicon. In this context, it is interesting to note that the Calcios preparation recommended by Cayce also supplies magnesium, phosphorus, and trace minerals including iodine, which supports metabolic function by strengthening the thyroid.

Chromium.   Chromium is a trace mineral that plays a critical role in normal carbohydrate metabolism. It supports the function of insulin and is also involved in the synthesis of fatty acids, cholesterol, and amino acids. Research findings strongly suggest that dietary chromium has a stabilizing effect on abnormal blood sugar conditions. Chromium is found in whole grains and brewer's yeast and, in smaller amounts, is also present in meat, cheese, and egg yolks.

Although required by the body in infinitesimal amounts, this mineral is often deficient in the diet, particularly in North America, where grains and flour products are predominantly refined. The condition is severely aggravated by a chronic deficiency of chromium in our agricultural soils. A high intake of refined sugars may further erode chromium levels in the body.

A deficiency in this mineral might be signaled by depressed growth or an inability to utilize glucose. A natural food-based supplement such as brewer's yeast, which also contains other nutrients that support the function of chromium in the body, helps to replenish chromium stores. Brewer's yeast is available in natural food stores in powder or tablet form.

Iodine.   An essential trace mineral, iodine is a vital constituent of the hormones produced by the thyroid gland. The thyroid controls several biochemical reactions, including oxygen utilization, protein synthesis, and the rate at which the body burns food.

Since ocean water contains iodine, most seafoods, edible seaweeds, and unrefined sea salt are good dietary sources of this mineral. Other iodine-rich foods include asparagus, watercress, Swiss chard, turnip greens, and dried beans; but their iodine content is determined by the presence or absence of this mineral in the soil in which they are grown. The iodine content of soil is typically low in bioregions located away from oceans.

An iodine deficiency can manifest in an endemic goiter, which is an enlargement of the thyroid gland, or in hypothyroidism, with possible symptoms such as chronic weight problems, cold hands and feet, and dry, brittle hair and nails.

An easy way to ensure sufficient iodine intake is by supplementation with kelp tablets or powder. This sea vegetable is an excellent natural source of iodine and other minerals. Kelp salt is recommended in the Cayce readings as a seasoning and substitute for common table salt.

Another form of iodine often recommended by Cayce for purification and balancing of the endocrine system is Atomidine, an aqueous solution of iodine from iodine trichloride, which was said to be less toxic than other iodine supplements. In reading 358-2 Cayce says: *"... this [the Atomidine] will not only be a curative property, but a* preventative! *May be used internally and externally as well, and especially for any form of disorder in glands or tissue of body.*"

Although Atomidine is available in health food stores without prescription for external use and dental hygiene, it is legally a prescription item when taken internally, due to its high potency. Atomidine should not be taken in excessive doses and never at the same time as other iodine supplements, like kelp tablets, or any other multivitamin/mineral supplement containing iodine.

Dr. William A. McGarey believes that Atomidine is quite safe when taken in moderation. In his May 1997 health column in *Venture Inward* magazine, McGarey writes about taking Atomidine for glandular regeneration: "At our A.R.E. Clinic [in Phoenix, Arizona], we have suggested drinking one drop in a half glass of water the very first thing on a Monday morning; two drops on Tuesday; three drops on Wednesday; four on Thursday; and five on Friday. Then leave off on the weekend. Don't be concerned that you've been taking it too long. I've been using it for forty years."

Iron.   Present in the body in small amounts, iron plays a major role in human growth and health maintenance. Iron is a vital component of hemoglobin, the oxygen carrier in the blood. It is also involved in energy production, protein metabolism, and normal brain function.

Dietary iron is obtained from meats, fish, eggs, green leafy vegetables, legumes, and dried fruit. It is also found in black cherries, some types of berries, seeds, whole grains, and sea vegetables. Pyridoxine (vitamin B_6) and ascorbic acid (vitamin C) promote iron utilization. Only a small percentage of dietary iron is actually absorbed by the body. So-called "heme" iron (from meat sources) is more readily absorbed than non-heme iron (from plant sources). Iron requirements are significantly increased in pregnant and lactating women.

Tiredness, lethargy, and shortness of breath are some of the symptoms associated with iron deficiency anemia.

When Cayce recommended an iron supplement, he frequently favored a liquid tonic containing beef extract and red wine. This specific product, Wyeth Beef and Wine, is no longer available today. Effective alternatives are herbal iron supplements, available in liquid form at health food stores, which are easily digested and absorbed. Certain herbs, such as red raspberry leaves and yellow dock, also supply readily assimilable iron.

Magnesium. In a society stressed to the limit, magnesium takes on major importance through its role in supporting the health of the nervous system. It assists enzyme function and facilitates the metabolism of calcium and phosphorus. Magnesium is essential for normal growth, protein synthesis, and energy production. It also acts as a cofactor in the function of the B-complex vitamins.

Magnesium is found in chlorophyll-rich green vegetables, whole grains, legumes, honey, molasses, dates, and nuts, especially almonds, cashews, and brazil nuts. Fish and sea kelp are also good sources.

An extensive body of research suggests that low magnesium levels are linked to heart disease, high blood pressure, and irregular heartbeat. Other known deficiency symptoms include nervousness, depression, and mental confusion. In addition, weakness, muscle tremor and spasm, and lack of coordination may be indicative of inadequate magnesium intake. Concentrated chlorophyll, in liquid or tablet form, is a natural supplement of magnesium.

Phosphorus. Next to calcium, phosphorus is the second most abundant mineral in the human body. Some 80 percent of it is found in the bones and teeth. The remainder is distributed throughout the nerves and muscle tissue. Phosphorus is closely related to calcium, and the two minerals function most effectively in a 1:2 ratio in the body. Phosphorus plays an important role in fat metabolism, protein synthesis, and energy production. It is required for cell growth and tissue repair and as an activator for the B-complex vitamins. Phosphorus is a cofactor of many enzymes and assists in maintaining the proper acid/alkaline balance in the body.

Phosphorus is abundant in a natural foods diet, which includes whole grains, nuts, legumes, eggs, meats, fish, and poultry. Milk also supplies phosphorus, but, according to Cayce, only when the milk is fresh and unpasteurized. Cayce also pointed to root vegetables and mentioned carrots, celery, turnips, and parsnips as good sources of phosphorus. The almond, mentioned as a medicinal food in many readings (see chapter 5), was singled out in one reading as carrying *"more phosphorus and iron in a combination easily assimilated than any other nut."* (1131-2) The readings advised against taking phosphorus in a synthetic preparation, which was said to be difficult to absorb.

Although a phosphorus deficiency in humans is uncommon, it can develop with the long-term use of antacids, which interfere with phosphorus absorption. As with calcium, vitamin D is required for the absorption of phosphorus, and a lack of this vitamin may deplete phosphorus levels. Symptoms of insufficient phosphorus include defective teeth and gums, fragile bones, and nervous conditions.

Overconsumption of phosphorus, which is possible through excessive amounts of meats, carbonated soft drinks, and convenience foods, may interfere with calcium metabolism and also deplete magnesium.

Potassium.　Potassium is essential for controlling intracellular fluids and the acid/alkaline balance in the body. It is involved in various metabolic processes, as well as in nerve transmission and muscle contraction. Potassium regulates the heartbeat and stimulates peristaltic action in the intestinal tract. It also helps to maintain cellular integrity and water balance.

Potassium is found abundantly in food sources, occurring in vegetables, fruits, whole grains, nuts, legumes, molasses, meats, and seafoods. Two potassium-rich foods, figs and dates, are the main ingredients in Mummy Food, recommended in the Cayce readings (see chapter 5).

A potassium deficiency can manifest as muscle weakness, nervousness, insomnia, diminished or irregular heartbeat, excessive thirst, and, in severe cases, even in respiratory failure. These conditions may be experienced as a result of prolonged diarrhea and/or vomiting, or anything else that might precipitate a state of dehydration, such as the long-term use of laxatives and diuretic medications. Long-term fasts can also upset potassium levels and should therefore only be undertaken with professional guidance. A healthy person who eats a well-balanced natural foods diet is unlikely to experience a potassium deficiency.

Zinc. Although zinc, an essential trace mineral, is required in only minute concentrations throughout the body, it is of vital importance for developmental growth and wound healing. Zinc plays a major role in protein metabolism and is required for healthy skin and hair and for proper immune function. The male reproductive organs also depend on adequate dietary intake of zinc.

Zinc occurs in whole grains, mushrooms, sunflower seeds, and whole grain products. Meats, egg yolks, and some seafoods, particularly herring and oyster, are also good sources of this mineral.

Refined, processed foods are the major robbers of dietary zinc.

Deficiency symptoms include retarded growth and

delayed sexual maturity, sterility, poor appetite, slow wound healing, and loss of taste and smell. Brewer's yeast is an excellent food-source supplement of zinc.

7

Nutritional Needs of Special Times and Circumstances

In meeting the needs, then, of the physical conditions of this body—first consideration must be of a diet in accord with the *developments* of the conditions existent, and the vibratory forces as would be changed in same should be in accord *with* the diet . . .

5603-1

OUR NUTRITIONAL NEEDS change as we change. They are influenced by our activities, our lifestyles, and our attitudes. The athlete who pursues competitive sports cannot perform well on a diet that is adequate for someone who spends many hours each day behind a desk in sedentary activity. Vegetarians and meat eaters must pay attention to specific aspects of their respective diets. Unquestionably, young children have needs that differ from those of mature adults.

At no other time is nutrition as important as during key

stages of growth and development. By recognizing and meeting the special needs of the body during such times, we can be assured of a lifetime of good health, free of the complaints typically associated with life's developmental stages.

Optimal Nutrition in Pregnancy

Pregnancy is a perfectly natural process, one which the healthy female body is designed to cope with. But unless a woman supports her body during this important time with optimal nutrition, as well as adequate rest and exercise, her health and that of her child may be compromised.

Research has shown that the diet of both parents prior to conception is a determining factor in the development of a healthy fetus. The health of a man's sperm is strongly influenced by good nutrition. A natural foods diet rich in fruits and vegetables, along with appropriate supplementation, ideally from whole-foods concentrates, can also help to prepare a woman's body for conception and child bearing, as well as avoid many of the discomforts commonly experienced in pregnancy.

The first trimester, especially, is a challenging time for many women. Hormonal changes often cause nausea, sometimes accompanied by a change in taste perception. So-called "morning sickness" is not necessarily restricted to mornings. Trying to eat well while feeling nauseous is not easy. Cayce often recommended an antinausea formula consisting of limewater and cinnamonwater, sometimes in combination with potassium bromide and potassium iodide. Unfortunately, this formula is no longer commercially available. Additional remedies suggested by Cayce are lime juice, orange juice, or freshly squeezed grape juice. The occasional use of Coca-Cola syrup[1] in noncarbonated water was also recommended.

Other effective natural remedies for nausea experienced during pregnancy include ginger root powder, taken as a tea or in capsule form, and the vitamin B complex, notably vitamin B$_6$. *Ipecac* and *Nux Vomica* are commonly prescribed homeopathic remedies.

In her diet, a pregnant woman must pay special attention to adequate protein. Proteins are the building blocks of body cells and are very important for the growing fetus. Inadequate protein intake can cause excessive fatigue, muscle weakness, and increased susceptibility to infection. Fish, fowl, eggs, milk, yogurt, and cheese are excellent protein sources. For vegetarians, combinations of legumes with either whole grains, nuts, or seeds offer complete plant protein. These may be difficult to digest for some, especially during pregnancy, when the digestive system does not always function at an optimal level. Nonmeat eaters who are allergic to eggs or dairy or who prefer to avoid them for other reasons may be well advised to consult a naturopathic physician, qualified nutritionist, or other knowledgeable health professional. An excellent all-vegetarian protein supplement, which also supplies numerous other nutrients, is *spirulina*, a cultivated fresh water algae.

A diet rich in vitamins and minerals is most important. Pregnant women have increased requirements for all nutrients, but especially for iron, calcium, folic acid, and zinc. Cayce emphasized such vegetables as lettuce, carrots, celery, cabbage, and squash in his dietary recommendations for pregnant women. One or more of the natural whole-food concentrates mentioned in chapter 5 can help to ensure that any important nutrients lacking in the diet are supplied in balance. In pregnancy, blood volume increases by 50 percent and the fetus builds up iron stores, so a good iron supplement becomes indispensable. The liquid, herbal-based iron formulations available in health food stores are highly effective and do not cause constipation, as is common with their pharmaceutical counterparts.

Calcium is important for bone and tooth development. The growing fetus draws large amounts of calcium from the mother, so adequate intake in pregnancy must be ensured. Although dairy products are a good source of calcium, this mineral is more readily assimilated from chlorophyll-rich dark-green vegetables, such as broccoli, kale, and watercress. Chlorophyll is high in magnesium, essential for the proper utilization of calcium.

As seen in the preceding chapter, Cayce recommended eating carrots, turnips, and the soft ends of chicken bones for extra dietary calcium. Calcios, Cayce's preferred calcium supplement, was especially recommended for pregnant women. Calcios is easily assimilated, which is important during pregnancy when digestive capacity may be impaired. In reading 951-7, Cayce suggested: *"Calcios is the better manner to take calcium. It is more easily assimilated, and will act better with pregnancy than any type of calcium products as yet presented."*

Folic acid, a member of the B-complex vitamins, builds blood, aids normal cell growth, and has been shown to prevent neural tube defects in infants. Whole grains, yeast, and dark leafy greens are good food sources of this important nutrient. Cabbage and orange juice, both recommended by Cayce, also supply folic acid.

Zinc is an important mineral for proper growth and development; therefore, inadequate levels during pregnancy increase the risk of spontaneous abortion, toxemia, and prolonged labor. Maternal deficiency can also result in retarded fetal growth and presents a greater risk of malformation. Good food sources of zinc include milk, meat, and egg yolks. Whole grains and cereal also supply zinc.

Essential fatty acids are important for the healthy development of the baby's brain and nervous system. Many modern diets are deficient in this nutrient, so supplementation during pregnancy is recommended. Flaxseed oil, borage oil, and oil of evening primrose supply the types of fatty acids most often missing in the diet. Without question, pregnancy is one of the most challenging times in a woman's life. With appropriate dietary adjustments, a suitable exercise program, and a positive attitude toward her body, her baby, and the amazing creative process in which she is privileged to partake, pregnancy can also become the most rewarding of times.

Giving Baby the Best Nutritional Start

Children are "the hope of the world," say the Cayce readings. Those of us who are parents have the responsibility of ensuring that our children's needs are met—physically, emotionally, and spiritually. When a soul enters a new body at birth, the physical need appears to dominate. The baby, who knew no hunger or thirst while in the womb, now needs food.

Nothing meets this need more completely than breast milk, which is nature's perfect infant formula. Right from the start, it provides baby with the full spectrum of nutrients necessary to support optimal growth and development. Breast milk supplies all necessary amino acids, vitamins, minerals, enzymes, and other nutrients in an easily digestible, optimally assimilable form. Powerful immunoglobulins, leukocytes, and other infection-fighting agents in breast milk offer protection against viruses and bacteria. There is evidence that breastfeeding protects against allergies, meningitis, respiratory and intestinal infections, and sudden infant death syndrome. It also lowers the infant's risk of developing juvenile diabetes and childhood lymphoma. Both the incidence and severity of colds and ear infections are significantly reduced in breastfed infants.

Breast milk further promotes the colonization of "friendly" lactobacillus bifidus in the baby's intestines, preventing harmful bacteria, such as those that cause severe diarrhea, from settling in. The healthy colon flora thus created is essential for the proper absorption and assimilation of nutrients.

Mother's milk contains white blood cells, which act like scavengers in the baby's intestines to identify and destroy harmful bacteria. In addition, infection-fighting immunoglobulins present in breast milk provide immune protection at a time when a baby's immature immune system is still developing. Both white blood cells and immunoglobulins are abundant in colostrum, the special first milk produced in the hours and days immediately following birth.

The bioavailability of nutrients found in breast milk is enhanced by special enzymes such as lactoferrin, which assists in the transport of iron. The iron found in breast milk is more readily absorbed than that from formula or iron-fortified baby foods. Breastfed infants are less likely to suffer from iron deficiency, especially if other liquids or foods are not offered at the same time as breast milk, since they can interfere with iron absorption.

Zinc, important for proper growth and development, is also better absorbed from breast milk than from formula. A zinc-binding protein contained in breast milk increases absorption in the baby's intestinal tract. Soy-based formulas, particularly, put infants at risk for a deficiency of zinc and other minerals, because phytates contained in soy have an inhibitory effect on the absorption of minerals.

Mother's milk is an ideal brain food, too. It contains cholesterol, which is vital for the growth and development of the brain and nervous system. Cholesterol is also a precursor of important hormones and is required for the formation of vitamin D and bile. A number of essential fatty acids, notably the omega-3 group of fats, also play a significant role in enhancing brain growth. Children who were breastfed as infants have been shown to have higher intelligence quotients as compared to formula-fed children.

Commercial infant formulas cannot duplicate all of the unique constituents of breast milk. The readings' viewpoint regarding synthetically formulated nutrients—*"Nature is much better yet than science"* (759-13)—is particularly valid when feeding baby. It is estimated that breast milk contains at least 400 nutrients, including hormones and specific growth factors, not found in formula.

One inimitable feature of breast milk is its ability to change and adapt to the growing infant's needs. Throughout the baby's development, the biological responsiveness of mother's milk ensures prompt delivery of the right concentrations of nutrients with each nursing. During the first six months of the baby's life, for instance, the fat content of mother's milk is at its highest, supplying the caloric intake required to enhance rapid growth. The fat content subsequently drops, but continues to self-adjust daily, even within the course of a single feeding. Even antibodies to specific pathogens are delivered whenever the mother's immune system detects these in her environment or in the baby's saliva as it comes in contact with the nipple.

The health benefits of breastfeeding are undisputed today. Lactation experts recommend that babies be breastfed exclusively for at least six months and that, even after the introduction of solid foods, breastfeeding be continued for a considerable length of time. This recommendation is backed by the Innocenti Declaration on the Protection, Promotion, and Support of Breastfeeding, adopted in 1990 by the World Health Organization and UNICEF. The Innocenti Declaration advocates that children be breastfed for up to two years and beyond.

In North America, where an estimated 70 percent of babies are bottle-fed by the time they are four months old, the idea of a toddler still nursing is often considered unacceptable. Even mothers of newborns frequently lack the professional and social support required to establish a successful breastfeeding relationship with their babies. Many new mothers switch to formula feeding because they erroneously believe that they are not producing enough milk. Without the help of an experienced lactation consultant or midwife, who can teach proper latch-on and feeding techniques, most breastfeeding attempts stand little chance of success.

The Cayce readings suggest that the general health and nutritional status of the mother are of paramount importance in ensuring a good supply of nourishing milk for the baby. Like Cayce, nutritionally oriented lactation experts today recommend plenty of yellow and dark-green leafy vegetables as well as high-quality proteins and fats for the nursing mother. Brewer's yeast and the herbs blessed thistle, raspberry leaf, nettle, and fennel are natural supplements that have traditionally been employed to replenish important nutrients in lactating women.

A daily supplement of cold-pressed flaxseed oil ensures an adequate supply of the important omega-3-type fatty acids. Flaxseed oil has also been shown to increase milk supply.

Milk production is regulated by the endocrine system, which responds not only to good nutrition, but also to mental attitudes and emotions. The milk ejection reflex kicks in faster when the mother is relaxed. Cayce said that anger causes poisons to be secreted from the glands, pointing out that *"a nursing mother would find that an-*

ger would affect the mammary glands." (281-54) The readings indicate that purification of the glands with Atomidine might be helpful in preparing the mother's body for the demanding task of nursing a baby. In some instances, Cayce found the mother's glandular system to be so imbalanced that he deemed it necessary to advise against breastfeeding altogether.

While breastfeeding can be demanding in terms of the mother's time and energy, it offers many rewards. It not only benefits the physical and emotional health of the child, but also that of the mother: Women who breastfeed for extended periods of time enjoy a reduced risk of breast and ovarian cancer, as well as protection against osteoporosis and hip fractures in later life.

Nourishing Foods for Tiny Tots

Pediatricians recommend solid foods for formula-fed babies after four months, but for breastfed babies only after six. Evidently, breast milk provides more complete nourishment that does not need to be "supplemented" with solids prematurely. Some breastfed babies refuse solid foods much longer, for eight months up to a year. It is better not to force solids, but to offer them occasionally and see if they are accepted.

The digestive system of the infant is immature and sensitive. In contrast to popular baby-feeding practices, cereals are not an ideal first food. Amylase, the enzyme needed to digest the starch in grains, is not manufactured by the pancreas until the molar teeth are fully developed, which can be as late as twenty-four to thirty-six months. Babies do produce the enzymes required to digest proteins and fats. The lactose-digesting enzyme *lactase* is also present, suggesting that the milk-sugar contained in breast milk is the only source of carbohydrates suitable for a baby. This is a physiological fact disregarded by pediatricians (and parents) who are influenced by the aggressive advertising campaigns of baby cereal producers. Many nutrition experts believe that the early feeding of grains is at the root of many allergies, colic, and skin rashes caused by the fermentation of incompletely digested starches.

One of the best first solids that can safely be given to a baby is the yolk from a soft-boiled egg. Ideally, this would be a yolk high in omega-3 essential fatty acids, which are found in eggs laid by free-range flax-fed hens. The egg white, which is difficult to digest, should be removed. Egg yolks are a good source of complete protein and iron, as well as the important vitamins A, D, and B complex, including B_{12}. They also contain cholesterol, essential for brain development. Organic yogurt, kefir, and blended or sieved cottage cheese are other options.

A good way to introduce vegetables is in the form of broths, soups, or freshly pressed juices, in a 50/50 dilution with pure water. To the young baby, they should be offered by the spoonful, in small quantities at first, then gradually increased. Only one new food should be introduced at a time, with intervals of several days, so that any possible allergic reactions can be promptly identified. Fresh, ripe fruit may be prepared in the same way, or puréed and blended.

A fruit often recommended for babies is mashed banana, which contains a significant amount of amylase and thus almost digests itself. The Cayce readings are divided on bananas, however. Some people were told not to eat them at all, while others were advised to eat them only when naturally ripened and grown in the environment where the person lived. Few of us reside in locales where bananas are cultivated, and ripe bananas are difficult to find, since the varieties available in supermarkets are nearly always artificially ripened through gassing. Organic bananas are a possible alternative, but

SEEKING INFORMATION ON

**holistic health, spirituality, dreams,
intuition or ancient civilizations?
Call 1-800-723-1112, visit our Web site,
or mail in this postage-paid card for a FREE
catalog of books and membership information.**

Name: _____

Address: _____

City: _____

State/Province: _____

Postal/Zip Code: _____ Country: _____

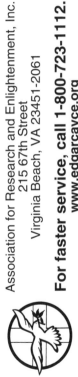

Association for Research and Enlightenment, Inc.
215 67th Street
Virginia Beach, VA 23451-2061

**For faster service, call 1-800-723-1112.
www.edgarcayce.org**

PBIN

they, too, are not always fully ripe.

Do not overtax the system with bananas, unless these are ripened in their natural state; for the activity of these in the beginnings of their deterioration—before they are palatable—makes for a hardship upon the system. But those that are overripe, or that have been gathered or prepared when they have fully matured, may be taken in moderation at certain meals or times. 658-15

At twelve months, some cooked fish and organic fowl, as well as cooked vegetables mashed with butter, may be added to the diet. Many parents may find it difficult to avoid cereals and other starches completely in the second year of their child's life. One way to make grains and cereals more digestible is to soak them for twenty-four hours and then cook them thoroughly. This initiates the breakdown of the carbohydrates and neutralizes phytates, which would otherwise inhibit mineral absorption.

Cayce consistently emphasized the importance of cooking grains well. In reading 1208-14, given for a two-and-a-half-year-old boy suffering from a bad cold and high fever, he recommended a fruit juice diet alternated with *"oatmeal,* preferably that *in the form of* cut *oats— not rolled oats—but this cooked for several hours in a double boiler."* Like many of the children who were presented to Cayce, this little boy was not well. However, the advice to cook the oats for several hours is one that everyone would do well to follow.

In a reading for a one-year-old baby girl, Cayce was asked what the child should be fed besides a commercial baby food. Cayce replied:

Any foods that are of easy digestion. Tomato

juice—especially that of canned tomatoes, that are canned good. Tomato juice or soups that are with beans, peas, tomatoes, potatoes. Celery soup may be given when properly prepared—not with lot of fat meat in any—but any of those conditions that supply the proper building to the body are well for the body. Well for the body to cut teeth on carrots, or parsnips (raw, see?)—these may be given, just so chunks are not cut off and swallowed too much. Lettuce, celery—any of these raw may be given, as much as eaten by the developing child, see? Not prepared in any special way and manner, but as may be taken in small quantity by the one using same. 608-1

Baby foods prepared at home with fresh, organic ingredients are unquestionably preferable to the popular store-bought jars of canned infant foods. Commercial baby food is usually diluted with water, starch, and fillers. Some of these products also contain refined sugars and preservatives. The convenience of prepared baby foods is understandably tempting in view of today's fast-paced lifestyles. Health food stores and many supermarkets now carry naturally preserved, organic baby foods without additives. These are helpful to have on hand when time is short and baby is hungry. Cayce was not generally opposed to prepared baby foods; in fact, he recommended the Gerber brand in several readings.

For children, as for adults, the readings advocate a diet high in fruits and vegetables, supplemented by meats of fish, fowl, or lamb. In a reading for a six-year-old girl, Cayce said: *"In the diet keep fruits and vegetables as the greater part, though—of course—fish, fowl and lamb may be as a part of the diet for the strengthening."* (1490-3)

As much as can possibly be arranged, a child's diet should be free of refined sugars, fried and processed foods, and artificial coloring and flavoring agents. What we feed our babies and toddlers determines not only how well they will thrive in youth, but also how healthy and resistant to illness they will be as adults. Early food choices establish patterns of health and immunity that literally set the stage for a life of wellness or disease. They also influence learning ability and successful social interaction, two important qualities for the happy, prosperous life that we all want our children to have.

Power Nutrition for Teens

During the teenage years, nutritional requirements skyrocket once again. The years from puberty to adulthood are marked by tremendous skeletal growth and significant hormonal changes. The endocrine system is thrown into overdrive, triggering much of the stress and upheavals typically associated with teenage life.

This is a time for superior nutrition in the form of high-quality protein, minerals, vitamins, enzymes, and important fatty acids. Ironically, many teenagers today subsist on diets of processed fast foods, such as french fries, hot dogs, donuts, candy bars, and sugared soft drinks laden with artificial flavoring and coloring agents.

Surveys have shown that female teenagers, in particular, are the most malnourished population segment in North America. It is hardly surprising, then, that many young women have weight, blood sugar, and skin problems. Incorrect or excessive dieting often makes the problem worse, sometimes resulting in obesity, anorexia, or bulimia.

The general Cayce diet, which emphasizes fruits, vegetables, and lean protein, is an ideal way to prevent or overcome the difficulties often attributed to hormonal changes. Teenagers also need to pay special attention to the growth minerals calcium, iron, and zinc. Calcium is needed for strong bones and healthy teeth, skin, hair, and nails. A teenager's rapid growth spurts make adequate calcium intake mandatory, as strong bone development during this period sets the stage for good bone health in later life. Incorporating more green leafy vegetables, orange juice, carrots, and turnips into the diet helps to boost calcium intake. Calcios, Cayce's calcium supplement of choice, should also be considered.

Iron plays a major role in growth and general health maintenance. Sports activities demanding a high degree of physical exertion, such as running, increase iron requirements. Studies indicate that all women of reproductive age are at risk for iron deficiency, and teenagers are no exception. If dietary iron from such foods as meat, eggs, green leafy vegetables, dried fruit, black cherries, whole grains, and sea vegetables does not meet the teenager's requirements, then a readily assimilable organic iron supplement, available in health food stores, can be helpful.

Requirements for zinc, important for reproductive organ development, especially in the male, rise during the teenage years. Zinc occurs in meat, egg yolks, mushrooms, sunflower seeds, whole grain products, and brewer's yeast. White spots appearing randomly on fingernails are considered to be a reliable indication of zinc deficiency.

Problem skin is the chief complaint among adolescents—some 80 percent of the teenage population suffers from acne to a greater or lesser extent. Due to hormonal changes, the oil glands become increasingly active, resulting in excess secretion and clogged pores. Although cleanliness and proper skin care are exceedingly important, the problem must be tackled from within.

Good digestion is a high priority for skin health. Sufficient dietary fiber from fruits, vegetables, and whole grains helps to prevent constipation. An excellent fiber supplement is the husk of psyllium seeds, available in health food stores. Drinking at least eight glasses of purified water daily, between meals, also promotes regularity. Vitamin A counts as an important skin nutrient. Best dietary sources are egg yolks, dairy products, liver, and fish liver oil. Carotenoids, the precursor form of vitamin A, are found in yellow, orange, and dark-green vegetables. To counteract deficiencies, especially when skin problems are present, it is advisable to supplement the diet with fish liver oil.

Stress can wreak havoc with skin, and the transition to adulthood is known to present its share of stressful challenges. Anxiety, nervous disorders, and depression occur with increasing frequency among the teenage population. The B-complex vitamins, with their nerve-building properties, have emerged as a popular antistress formula. Cayce often emphasized the yellow or orange vegetables as the best sources for B vitamins. Leafy greens, whole grains, and brewer's yeast also supply the B complex. Folic acid, a member of the B complex, is especially important for women of reproductive age. Studies have shown that some 40 percent of normally active adolescent girls are folic-acid deficient.

Junk food, soft drinks, and candy bars can't build a healthy body, but a diet rich in alkalizing fruits, vegetables, and lean protein can. For those on the threshold of adulthood, good nutrition has no substitute. A properly nourished teenager is far less likely to develop cravings for alcohol, drugs, or cigarettes. By giving our teens the best that nutritional science has to offer, we make an important contribution to building a healthy society.

Balancing Weight with the Cayce Diet

More than one third of Americans are considered to be overweight. Nearly half of all women and a quarter of all men in the United States are trying to lose weight at any given time, mainly through diet and exercise. Weight-loss programs and diet clubs are big business. For many dieters, their current attempt at achieving weight loss is not their first. Some have lost and regained their weight numerous times, each time ending up in worse condition and more discouraged than the last. Is there a way to break this cycle?

The reason most weight-loss diets fail is simple: They end up starving an already malnourished body. Whether we are seriously overweight or just in need of shedding a few extra pounds, the excess weight we carry is in direct proportion to the amount of nutrients that have not been supplied to the body or have not been assimilated. Genetic disposition and environmental factors come into play, but even these are influenced by our food choices.

Simply eating less is not the answer. Severely restricting food intake further deprives the body of nutrients. What is needed is an emphasis on quality, not quantity, of food. Put away the bathroom scale and stop counting calories. Choose nutrient-dense foods that will assist the body in its efforts to detoxify, nourish, and rebuild damaged cells. A healthy body will always balance its own weight. Individuals whose metabolism is seriously impaired may need professional help in selecting a personalized nutrition program that addresses their unique biochemical requirements. But anyone can benefit from following the basic principles of healthy eating, compatible with the Cayce approach:

1. Drink six to eight glasses of filtered, distilled, or spring

water each day. Really do it! Water is needed for proper eliminations, to flush out toxins, and to deliver nutrients to the cells. Sip small amounts throughout the day.

2. Eat a vegetable-based diet. Mentally reverse the outdated concept of vegetables as a side dish on your dinner plate. Make vegetables the center of your meals, and always include at least one dark-green leafy and one yellow- or orange-colored vegetable. Limit root and pod vegetables to one per meal. Eat at least one third of your veggies raw, and prepare others by steaming, baking, or cooking them in parchment paper to preserve nutrients. The vitamins, minerals, fiber, enzymes, phytochemicals, and nutraceuticals in vegetables aid in balancing the body's metabolism. Eat six to eight servings of vegetables a day, more if you like, giving priority to the green leafy types. It is difficult to overeat on vegetables!

3. Eat a serving of high-quality protein two or three times a day. Protein is required for proper metabolic function and endocrine balance. Fish, fowl, egg yolks, and dairy products (ideally fermented, such as yogurt) provide excellent protein. Vegetarian sources are combinations of legumes, grains, seeds, and nuts. Avoid red meat. And never fry or deep-fry fish, fowl, or any other food.

4. Avoid excessive intake of starches, especially processed carbohydrates and white-flour products. These are "empty calories" and nutrient robbers that cause weight gain in the first place. White bread, donuts, pastries, and candy bars create drosses in the system. Cayce warned of mixing quantities of sweets and starches at the same time. Reading 1040-1, given for a woman who complained of excessive weight gain, says: *"Remember that the acids are formed in too great quantities through*

excess quantities of starches (as potatoes or white breads or the like) with *quantities of sweets."* According to Cayce, an excess of starches in the diet has a detrimental effect on endocrine function, creating a state of glandular imbalance. A good rule of thumb is to serve no more than one starchy food with each meal. If you like potatoes, eat them, but not at the same meal as rice or bread. Give preference to unrefined grain products, such as brown rice and whole wheat.

5. Satisfy cravings for sweets by eating a small amount of raw honey or some ripe fruit. Grapes, in particular, are ideal for any weight-loss program. They have a cleansing effect on the system, promoting good digestion and assimilation, as well as glandular coordination. Grape juice, diluted 2:1 with water, taken before meals and at bedtime, is repeatedly recommended in the Cayce readings for individuals suffering from obesity.

6. Avoid refined, processed, or hydrogenated fats, such as those found in margarine and commercial vegetable oils. These interfere with the function of essential fatty acids, important for metabolic health. The Cayce-recommended fats—butter and olive oil [extra virgin]—may be taken in moderation. Eliminating fats completely can seriously disrupt metabolic function and ultimately sabotage an attempt to lose weight. But the right choice of fat is important.

7. Supplement your diet with a green-food concentrate and a reliable source of iodine, such as ocean kelp or Atomidine, to be taken periodically as recommended by Cayce. Iodine is a vital nutrient for the thyroid, which controls numerous metabolic functions, including the rate at which the body burns food.

8. Eat only when hungry, and only until full. Eat in a relaxed atmosphere, and chew all food thoroughly.

Followed consistently, the Cayce diet will promote any weight loss that is needed by the body. Wrong food choices are what caused those extra pounds to accumulate. The right food choices will help the body find its proper weight. Regular exercise, a positive mental outlook, and a dose of patience will do the rest.

The Vegetarian Diet

When asked by a vegetarian whether she should continue to follow her meatless diet, Cayce replied: *"This from the material angle is not an absolute necessity—but in all good conscience, keep that as thy soul (we didn't say heart)—thy soul—desires."* (1554-6)

Today, vegetarianism is more popular than ever in our Western society. Encouraged by research findings which consistently demonstrate that vegetarians are at considerably lower risk for serious health conditions such as heart disease, stroke, high blood pressure, cancer, and diabetes, a growing number of individuals are seeking to replace their daily meat servings with healthier alternatives. Eating lower on the food chain, vegetarians minimize the dangers of ingesting concentrated amounts of poisonous chemicals, hormones, and antibiotic residues often found in meat.

The ethical and environmental considerations of a vegetarian lifestyle are equally significant. In the Yogic tradition, the practice of *ahimsa* (nonviolence) through a vegetarian diet has long been considered essential for spiritual growth and the evolution of consciousness. In contrast, large-scale factory farming operations, which often subject animals to much suffering during their short, unhappy lives destined to end violently at the slaughterhouse, are also major contributors to environmental pollution and destruction. It takes considerably less land and water to produce a vegetarian's primarily plant-based diet than to raise livestock for food consumption. The future of our planet Earth, as well as the lives of millions of its inhabitants, may depend on our willingness to substantially reduce meat intake and thus share the available natural resources with those less affluent.

By recommending minimal amounts of meat, fowl, and fish, the Cayce readings go a long way toward achieving this objective. Cayce's dietary guidelines, with their strong emphasis on natural foods and fresh fruits and vegetables, were years ahead of their time and even today require considerable lifestyle changes of those switching from a typical meat-and-potato or convenience-food diet.

The opinions of experts are divided on whether or not animal products are necessary in the normal diet. A concern often raised is that the vegetarian diet does not supply adequate protein. The word protein is derived from the Greek *proteios*, which means *of first importance* and reflects the indispensable status of protein in nutrition. Proteins are composed of amino acids, most of which the body is able to manufacture from a variety of raw materials. There are, however, at least eight essential amino acids which must be obtained from the diet. All foods, including vegetables and fruit, contain some amino acids, but the ideal ratio of the eight essential ones is present only in meat, fowl, fish, eggs, and dairy products. By properly combining certain plant foods, such as grains and legumes, nuts or seeds, which complement each other's amino acid portfolio, it is possible to obtain complete protein even from a plant-based diet.

There are different types of vegetarians: *Lacto-ovo veg-*

etarians do not eat meat of any kind, but they do eat eggs and dairy. *Lacto vegetarians* eat dairy products but no eggs. *Vegans* eat no foods of animal origin whatsoever. Is it possible to be a vegetarian while following the Cayce diet? A lacto-ovo or lacto vegetarian who includes a variety of fruits and vegetables, whole grains, nuts, as well as some eggs and dairy in the diet, can stay well within the general Cayce guidelines. A vegan, who consumes more acid-forming grains, legumes, nuts, and seeds for protein, may find it more difficult to adhere to an 80 percent alkalizing diet.

Many vegetarians rely heavily on soybeans, which are higher in protein than other plant foods. Some nutrition researchers, however, are concerned that not all soy products are health promoting. Soybeans are high in phytates, which inhibit the absorption of essential minerals such as calcium, magnesium, iron, and zinc. The phytate content in traditionally fermented soy products, such as tempeh and miso, is reduced; but in the more popular tofu, made from soybean curd, phytates remain high. Research has shown that vegetarian diets high in soybean products may promote iron deficiency, particularly in women.

The Cayce readings mention soybeans infrequently. In one case, a questioner who asked what was the best meat substitute was told *"soy beans."* (257-252) In general, however, soy products are recommended with a caveat. They are said to be beneficial only for physically active individuals. When asked whether it was *"advisable for the body to drink* soy bean milk," Cayce replied: *"This will depend much upon the activities of the body. If there is sufficient of the energies used for physical activities to make same more easily assimilated, it is well. If these energies are used for activities which are more mental than physical, it would not be so well."* (1158-18)

In recent years, meatless diets have gained acceptance among mainstream nutritionists. A position paper released by the American Dietetic Association in 1997 states that a well-planned vegetarian diet which excludes all animal protein can be nutritionally adequate. Others disagree. Nutrition specialist Ann Louise Gittleman, who has authored several books on nutrition, quotes research by Don Tyson, former director of Aatron Medical Services in Hawthorne, California, which showed that plasma and urine tests in vegetarians consistently revealed a shortage of several amino acids, even though these people ate complementary plant protein.

This is consistent with research by the late Dr. Weston Price, who found that those consuming a diet which includes animal protein showed better growth rates and health patterns than those who relied primarily on plant foods for protein.

There is also evidence of great variation in the amino acid requirements among the general population. Individual biochemistry plays a significant role. Some individuals are unable to manufacture certain amino acids considered "nonessential" because most people's bodies can readily synthesize them. During times of stress and exertion, amino acid requirements can increase dramatically. This is reflected in Cayce's follow-up advice to the vegetarian woman whose reading was quoted above: *"Vegetables are nature's way, the natural, the correct, the cleansing. Keep it, then; but these are as to the needs of the self depending upon the manner of expending energies. So long as there is the expending of self in mental, yes. When it becomes active in great physical exertion—as it will, in the experience—then there will be the needs for some changes to be made."* (1554-6)

Nutritional needs can indeed vary considerably, not just from person to person, but also within the same individual, depending on circumstances and physiological developments.

There is no question that meat intake in our affluent Western society is excessive and that most people could reap dramatic benefits from significantly reducing their consumption of meat, especially red meat. A concomitant increase in the consumption of vegetables and fruit would no doubt reduce the incidence of heart disease, cancer, and other degenerative conditions.

Progressive nutrition researchers have theorized that the body's need for nutrients, including protein, decreases as it evolves in consciousness. In *Spiritual Nutrition and the Rainbow Diet,* Dr. Gabriel Cousins suggests that "as our system changes with meditation, fasting, eating lighter, and increasing raw food intake . . . the protein we take in moves into the cells more readily." This idea certainly deserves to be considered, especially in view of the fact that a more evolved state of being enables us to respond differently to stressful situations, whether they be physical, mental, or emotional. A positive stress response means better nutrient assimilation and conservation in the body.

Whether we choose a vegetarian lifestyle or prefer to include meat in the diet, the principles of the Edgar Cayce diet can assist us in preparing body and mind for the major shift in consciousness which is likely to be required of us as we move into the new millennium.

Notes

Chapter 1
1. Taken from *Diet for a New America,* by John Robbins.
2. The next chapter discusses how to maintain an alkaline/acid balance.
3. See the Resources section for guidelines on obtaining Patapar paper.
4. Gelatin is discussed in greater detail in chapter 5.
5. See the Resources section for guidelines on obtaining Coca Cola syrup.

Chapter 2
1. Those interested in more information on this subject may wish to obtain a copy of a 1997 study by the University of Illinois Department of Food Science and Human Nutrition, which showed that canned fruits and vegetables are nutritionally comparable to fresh and frozen. Chapter 4 discusses this in greater detail.
2. See the Resources section for help in obtaining pH-testing paper.
3. See the Resources section for guidelines on obtaining Glyco-Thymoline.

Chapter 3
1. Lactobacillus bulgaricus is a dairy culture used in yogurt making.

Chapter 4
1. Study by Prof. Bernhard H. Blanc, Institute for Biochemistry at the Swiss Technical College in Lausanne, and Dr. Hans U. Hertel of the Bio-environmental Research and Consultancy Center in Wattenwill, Switzerland.
   Reported in the *International Journal of Biosocial and Medical Research,* Volume 14, 1993.

Chapter 6
1. Calcidin is still compounded by a few pharmacists in

North America, but it must be prescribed first by a physician. For further help in obtaining this product, contact the A.R.E. Health and Rejuvenation Research Center, 757-428-7340.
2. The Resources section offers guidelines on obtaining hard-to-find items.
3. Not a true vitamin but considered a member of the B complex and an important cofactor in the function of B vitamins.
4. Not a true vitamin but considered a member of the B complex and an important cofactor in the function of B vitamins.
5. Not a true vitamin but considered a member of the B complex and an important cofactor in the function of B vitamins.

Chapter 7
1. Limewater, alone, is available; as is Coca-Cola syrup. See the Resources section for guidelines on obtaining these items.

References

Alkalize or Die
by Dr. Theodore A. Baroody
Eclectic Press, Waynesville, N.C.
An Edgar Cayce Encyclopedia of Foods for Health and Healing
compiled by Brett Bolton
A.R.E. Press, Virginia Beach, Va., 1997
An Edgar Cayce Home Medicine Guide
A.R.E. Press, Virginia Beach, Va., 1982
Ann Wigmore's Recipes for Longer Life
by Dr. Ann Wigmore
Avery Publishing Group, Inc., Wayne, N.J., 1978
Biological Transmutations
by Professor C. Louis Kervran
Happiness Press, Magalia, Calif., 1980
Butter Is Better
by Sally W. Fallon, M.A., and Mary G. Enig, Ph.D.
Health Freedom News, Nov./Dec., 1995
Butter, the Healthier Choice
by Zoltan P. Rona, M.D., M.Sc.
Health Naturally Magazine, Nov./Dec., 1992
Color, Light and Low Level Electromagnetic Radiation: Their Effects on Plants, Animals and People, Part 8
by John Nash Ott, Sc.D. (Hon.)
International Journal of Biosocial and Medical Research
Volume 14, 1993
Dian Dincin Buchman's Herbal Medicine: The Natural Way to Get Well and Stay Well
Gramercy Publishing Company, N.Y., 1980
Diet for a New America
by John Robbins
Stillpoint Publishing, Walpole, N.H., 1987
Enzyme Nutrition: The Food Enzyme Concept
by Dr. Edward Howell
Avery Publishing Group, Inc., Wayne, N.J., 1985
Fats That Heal, Fats That Kill
by Udo Erasmus
Alive Books, Burnaby, B.C., 1994

Fish Consumption and Risk of Sudden Cardiac Death
by Christine M. Albert, M.D.; Charles H. Hennekens, M.D.;
Christopher J. O'Donnel, M.D.; Umed A. Ajani, MBBS;
Vincent J. Carey, Ph.D.; Walter C. Willet, M.D.; Jeremy N.
Ruskin, M.D.; and JoAnn E. Manson, M.D.
Journal of the American Medical Assn., Vol. 279, No. 1, 1998
Fit for Life
by Harvey and Marilyn Diamond
Warner Books, Inc., New York, N.Y., 1985
Food and Healing
by Annemarie Colbin
Ballantine Books, New York, N.Y., 1996
Food Combining for Health
by Doris Grant and Jean Joyce
Healing Arts Press, Rochester, Vt., 1989
Foods That Heal
by Dr. Bernard Jensen
Avery Publishing Group, Inc., Garden City Park, N.Y., 1993
Healing Psoriasis: The Natural Alternative
by Dr. John O.A. Pagano
The Pagano Organization, Inc., Englewood Cliffs, N.J., 1991
Hiatal Hernia Syndrome: Insidious Link to Major Illness
by Dr. Theodore A. Baroody
Eclectic Press, Waynesville, N.C., 4th Printing, 1993
Honey as a Source of Antioxidants
by M. Berenbaum et al.
Journal of Apicultural Res., Vol. 37, pp. 221-225, 1998
How to Fight Cancer and Win
by William L. Fischer
Fischer Pub. Corp., Canfield, Ohio, 1994
*Kefir Rediscovered: The Nutritional Benefits of an Ancient
Health Food*
by Klaus Kaufmann
Alive Books, Burnaby, B.C., 1997
Light: Medicine of the Future
by Jacob Liberman, O.D., Ph.D.
Bear & Company Publishing, Santa Fe, N.M., 1991
Light, Radiation & You
by John N. Ott

Devin-Adair, Greenwich, Conn., 1990

Nourishing Traditions
by Sally Fallon, with Pat Connolly and Mary G. Enig, Ph.D.
ProMotion Publishing, San Diego, Calif., 1995

Nourishing Wisdom: A Mind/Body Approach to Nutrition and Well-Being
by Marc David
Bell Tower, New York, N.Y., 1991

Nourishment Home Grown: How to Grow Real Nutritious Foods in Your Back Yard
by Dr. Alexander Beddoe
S. & J. Unlimited, Oroville, Wash., 1992

Nutrient Conservation in Canned, Frozen and Fresh Foods
by Dr. Barbara P. Klein
University of Illinois Department of Food Science and Human Nutrition, 1997

Physician's Reference Notebook
by William A. McGarey, M.D.
A.R.E. Press, Virginia Beach, Va., 4th Printing, 1991

Skin Diseases
by Jan de Vries
Mainstream Publishing Company, Ltd., Edinburgh, U.K., 1992

Spiritual Nutrition and the Rainbow Diet
by Gabriel Cousins, M.D.
Cassandra Press, San Rafael, Calif., 1986

Systemic Enzyme Therapy
by Hector E. Solorzano del Rio, M.D., D.Sc., Ph.D.
Townsend Ltr. for Doctors, Vol. 76, May 1995

The Baby Book
by William Sears, M.D., and Martha Sears, R.N.
Little, Brown and Company, New York, N.Y., 1993

The Calcium Factor: The Scientific Secret of Health and Youth
by Robert R. Barefoot and Carl J. Reich, M.D.
Bokar Consultants (U.S.) Inc., Wickenburg, Ariz., 2nd Edition (revised), 1996

The Complete Edgar Cayce Readings for Windows (CD-ROM)
A.R.E. Press, Virginia Beach, Va., 1995

The Edgar Cayce Handbook for Health Through Drugless Therapy

by Dr. Harold J. Reilly and Ruth Hagy Brod
A.R.E. Press, Virginia Beach, Va., 1975
The Essene Gospel of Peace. Book One.
The Third-Century Aramaic Manuscript and Old Slavonic Texts
Compared, Edited, and Translated by Dr. Edmond Bordeaux Szekely
International Biogenic Society, Nelson, B.C., 1981
The Friendly Bacteria: How Lactobacilli and Bifidobacteria Can Transform Your Health
by William H. Lee, R.Ph., Ph.D.
Keats Publishing, Inc., New Canaan, Conn., 1988
The Healing Aspects of Honey
by Ross Conrad
Health Freedom News, July 1993
The Parents' Guide to Better Nutrition for Tots to Teens (And Others!)
by Emery W. Thurston, Ph.D., Sc.D.
Keats Publishing, New Canaan, Conn., 1979
The Power of Superfoods
by Sam Graci
Prentice Hall Canada, Inc., Scarborough, Ont., 1997
The Womanly Art of Breastfeeding
La Leche League International
Penguin Books, New York, N.Y., 1991
The Wonderful World of Bee Pollen
by Joe M. Parkhill
Country Bazaar Publishing Co., Berryville, Alaska, 1982
Trying the Apple Diet
by Bob Revay
Venture Inward Magazine, Nov./Dec. 1993
Vital Foods for Total Health
by Dr. Bernard Jensen
Bernard Jensen Products, Solano Beach, Calif., 1984

Resources

The Cayce remedies, with the exception of Calcidin (see Notes; chapter 6), are available at many health food stores. If you experience difficulty obtaining certain items in your area, contact one of the following:

The Heritage Store
314 Laskin Road
Virginia Beach, VA 23451
Phone: 757-428-0100
Toll free ordering: 1-800-TO-CAYCE   (800-862-2923)
Fax: 757-428-3632
Web site: www.caycecures.com
e-mail: heritage@caycecures.com

The Cayce Corner
A.R.E. Medical Clinic
4018 North 40th Street
Phoenix, AZ 85018
Phone: 604-955-9206
Web site: www.eigi.com/are
e-mail: areclinic@eigi.com

Baar Products, Inc.
P.O. Box 60
Downingtown, PA 19335
Phone: 610-873-4591
Toll free ordering: 800-269-2502
Web site: www.baar.com
e-mail: bbaar@baar.com

Holistic Nutrition Centre & Healing Service
Toronto, Canada
Toll free: 1-877-256-4333
Web site: www.holistic-nutrition.com
e-mail: mail@holistic-nutrition.com

Index

A

Acid xiv, 5, 12, 18, 19, 20, 22, 23, 24, 25, 26, 27, 28, 29, 30, 31, 32, 34, 55, 56, 57, 58, 64, 65, 66, 68, 69, 72, 73, 76, 77, 78, 79, 80, 89, 92, 97, 98, 112, 113, 114, 117, 119, 121, 125, 128, 129, 132, 133, 134, 137, 138, 139, 140, 142, 144, 147, 149
Acid- and Alkaline-Forming Foods Chart 21
Alcohol(ic) 11, 50, 141
Alfalfa 44, 106, 115
Alkaline xiv, 5, 18, 19, 20, 22, 23, 24, 26, 27, 28, 29, 30, 31, 32, 33, 34, 65, 92, 117, 118, 119, 124
Alkaline Reserve 18
Alkalinity xiv, 17, 18, 19, 20, 23, 24, 25, 27, 28, 29, 30, 31, 34, 43, 117
Allergic 38, 59, 83, 129, 136
Allergies 34, 48, 96, 131, 136
Almond Milk 83, 84
Almond Oil 84
Almonds 7, 82, 83, 84, 119, 123
Aluminum 59
Amino Acid(s) 7, 62, 82, 90, 106, 107, 112, 120, 131, 146, 148
Amylase 37, 40, 51, 135, 136
Anemia 40, 90, 94, 95, 96, 99, 123
Animal Protein 3, 5, 7, 18, 73, 148
Antacid(s) 32, 124
Antibiotic(s) 9, 16, 48, 89, 145
Antioxidant(s) 8, 70, 82, 85, 95, 98, 113, 114
Apple Diet 85, 86, 87
Apple(s) 71, 82, 83, 84, 85, 86, 87
Arthritis 72, 90, 95, 96, 107, 118
Asparagus 23, 121
Assimilation(s) 10, 12, 13, 28, 29, 37, 39, 45, 48, 59, 62, 64, 68, 80, 85, 87, 89, 91, 92, 94, 114, 118, 132, 144, 149
Atomidine 121, 122, 135, 144

Attitude(s) 13, 14, 15, 28, 34, 127, 131, 134
Ayurveda 13, 75

B

Babies 120, 133, 134, 135, 136, 139
Baby Food(s) 132, 137, 138
Bacon 8, 59, 71, 78
Baking and Broiling 57
B-Complex Vitamins 6, 48, 82, 87, 107, 110, 111, 123, 124, 130, 141
Beans 7, 45, 56, 57, 63, 80, 115, 119, 121, 138
Beef Juice 8, 87, 88, 89
Bee Pollen 96, 97, 107
Beer 11
Beta Carotene 17, 109, 110
Beverage(s) 11
Bifidobacteria 48, 49
Bile 32, 71, 109, 133
Bile Salts 8
Bioflavonoid(s) 6, 41, 85, 95, 113
Black Pepper 10, 58
Blood 8, 11, 17, 18, 20, 28, 29, 40, 43, 70, 96, 115, 117, 122, 129, 130
Blood-Building 8, 38, 95
Blood Sugar 99, 120, 139
Bone(s) 28, 89, 90, 91, 114, 115, 117, 119, 123, 124, 130, 140
Bread xv, 7, 11, 15, 25, 26, 37, 46, 63, 64, 65, 78, 79, 80, 94, 95, 143, 144
Breakfast 7, 8, 26, 57, 65, 78
Breastfeeding 131, 133, 134, 135
Breast Milk 131, 132, 133, 135
Brewer's Yeast 111, 120, 121, 126, 134, 141
Broccoli 64, 74, 113, 115, 130
Bromelain 39, 51
Butter 9, 58, 59, 68, 70, 73, 78, 79, 83, 137, 144
Buttermilk 47, 111

C

Caffeine 11, 12, 67, 119
Calcios 105, 119, 120, 130, 140
Calcium 6, 18, 28, 29, 30, 31, 32, 47, 48, 54, 60, 79, 82, 85, 90, 102, 105, 113, 114, 116, 117, 118, 119, 120, 123, 124, 129, 130, 139, 140, 147
Cancer 6, 8, 9, 17, 48, 50, 51, 54, 64, 68, 83, 85, 91, 95, 106, 135, 145, 149
Candida Albicans 48
Canned and Frozen Foods 60
Canning 23, 50, 54, 60
Carbohydrates 32, 37, 63, 70, 135, 137, 143
Carbonated Beverage(s) 11
Carotenoid(s) 6, 54, 68, 109, 110, 141
Carrot Juice 41, 42, 43
Carrot(s) 6, 17, 35, 38, 41, 42, 43, 44, 66, 76, 79, 90, 119, 124, 129, 130, 138, 140
Cayce Diet 4, 5, 7, 9, 10, 14, 15, 55, 75, 117, 118, 139, 142, 145, 147, 149
Cayenne 10, 58
Celery 6, 17, 41, 44, 77, 79, 124, 129, 138
Cellulase 37
Cereal(s) 7, 26, 57, 65, 77, 78, 79, 80, 83, 86, 102, 130, 135, 136, 137
Cheese(s) 9, 28, 46, 64, 119, 120, 129, 136
Chewing 12, 13, 32, 36, 37, 95, 119
Child(ren) 2, 48, 62, 85, 94, 120, 127, 128, 131, 133, 134, 135, 137, 138, 139
Chlorophyll 5, 6, 36, 38, 106, 123, 130
Cholesterol 8, 9, 38, 46, 48, 62, 68, 69, 70, 71, 95, 120, 132, 136
Chromium 7, 120, 121
Chronic Fatigue 48
Circulation 11, 27, 84, 113, 118
Circulatory System 10, 20
Citrus Fruit(s) 7, 25, 26, 41, 65, 77, 78, 79, 80, 113
Cleansing Diet(s) 24, 92
Coca-Cola Syrup 11, 128
Coffee 11, 12, 59, 66, 67, 74, 78, 79, 82, 86
Coffee Substitute(s) 12

Cold(s) 5, 19, 20, 25, 26, 34, 91, 96, 109, 112, 132, 137
Consciousness 4, 6, 14, 145, 149
Constipation 85, 130, 141
Cooked Food(s) 38, 39, 40, 45, 46, 54
Cooking 6, 23, 25, 44, 45, 54, 55, 56, 57, 58, 59, 71, 72, 106, 109, 137, 143
Cooking Utensils 59
Copper 18
Craving(s) 10, 13, 76, 97, 99, 141, 144
Cream 12, 66, 84, 102
Cultured Dairy Products 46, 111

D

Dairy Product(s) 9, 18, 37, 49, 71, 109, 111, 114, 119, 130, 141, 143, 146, 147
Date(s) 101, 102, 123, 125
Degenerative Disease 3, 5, 17, 69
Diabetes 96, 131, 145
Diabetic 97, 98, 99, 100
Diarrhea 39, 125, 132
Diet xiv, 2, 3, 4, 5, 6, 7, 9, 10, 13, 14, 15, 16, 18, 19, 20, 24, 27, 28, 30, 32, 33, 34, 36, 41, 43, 44, 46, 48, 49, 54, 55, 63, 64, 66, 67, 70, 71, 72, 73, 75, 76, 77, 79, 80, 83, 85, 89, 92, 93, 95, 96, 100, 101, 104, 105, 106, 107, 108, 109, 111, 115, 117, 118, 119, 120, 124, 125, 127, 128, 129, 131, 137, 138, 139, 140, 141, 142, 143, 144, 145, 146, 147, 148
Digestion 9, 10, 11, 12, 13, 19, 23, 24, 32, 33, 34, 36, 37, 38, 39, 45, 50, 63, 68, 71, 97, 107, 137, 140, 144
Digestive Enzymes 26, 33, 36, 37, 40, 49, 50, 119

E

E. Coli 39
Egg(s) 8, 9, 11, 15, 78, 107, 114, 115, 122, 124, 129, 136, 140, 146, 147
Egg Yolks 8, 109, 115, 119, 120, 125, 130, 136, 140, 141, 143
Elimination(s) 11, 43, 45, 80, 87, 91, 92, 102, 104, 143
Emotions 27, 33, 134
Enzyme Inhibitors 25, 44, 45, 57

Enzyme(s) 10, 12, 19, 36, 37, 38, 39, 40, 41, 42, 43, 44, 45, 46, 47, 49, 51, 52, 60, 69, 92, 97, 99, 105, 106, 107, 116, 123, 124, 131, 132, 135, 139, 143
Enzyme Supplements 39, 40
Epilepsy 86
Essene Bread 46
Essential Fatty Acid(s) 6, 8, 38, 50, 72, 131, 133, 136, 144

F

Fast(s) 24, 71, 85, 86, 93, 97, 125, 149
Fat(s) 7, 9, 18, 20, 23, 24, 30, 32, 37, 38, 43, 46, 49, 57, 59, 62, 68, 69, 70, 71, 73, 78, 82, 88, 95, 109, 110, 124, 133, 134, 135, 138, 144
Fat-Soluble Vitamin(s) 9, 68, 109
Fatty Acid(s) 10, 70, 72, 105, 107, 120, 131, 134, 139
Fetus 128, 129, 130
Fiber 7, 37, 55, 82, 85, 92, 99, 140, 141, 143
Fig(s) 79, 80, 101, 102, 125
Fish 7, 24, 57, 71, 72, 73, 77, 80, 95, 114, 122, 123, 124, 129, 137, 138, 143, 146
Fish Liver Oil(s) 109, 110, 114, 118, 141
Flaxseed Oil 131, 134
Flu 19, 91
Folic Acid 32, 62, 110, 111, 129, 130, 141
Food Combinations 25, 63, 64, 65, 67, 68
Food Combining 32, 62, 64, 65, 67
Food Guide Pyramid 5
Fowl 7, 24, 71, 73, 77, 79, 80, 129, 137, 138, 143, 146
Free Radicals 41, 69, 70, 98, 109, 113
Freezing 23, 60, 61
Fried Foods 26, 32
Fruit and Vegetable Juice(s) 41
Fruit(s) 1, 3, 5, 6, 7, 18, 20, 22, 23, 24, 25, 26, 35, 36, 37, 39, 44, 54, 55, 60, 61, 65, 67, 73, 74, 75, 76, 77, 78, 79, 80, 84, 92, 109, 111, 113, 116, 117, 118, 122, 125, 128, 136, 137, 138, 139, 140, 141, 144, 146, 147, 149

Frying 57, 58, 72

G

Gallstone(s) 71
Gastric Secretion(s) 9, 63, 66
Gelatin 10, 39, 89, 90, 91
Gland(s) 13, 20, 24, 27, 28, 29, 63, 64, 67, 89, 94, 118, 121, 122, 134, 135, 140
Glyco-Thymoline 31
Grain(s) 3, 5, 6, 8, 12, 18, 19, 25, 44, 45, 46, 51, 57, 58, 78, 120, 135, 136, 137, 143, 144, 146
Grape Diet 93
Grape Juice 91, 92, 93, 94, 128, 144
Grape Poultice(s) 93
Grape(s) 91, 92, 93, 94, 95, 144, 147
Green Beans 74
Green-Food Concentrate(s) 106, 115, 144
Green Vegetable(s) 6, 38, 77, 79, 106, 109, 118, 123, 130, 141

H

Heart Disease 8, 9, 10, 47, 68, 69, 70, 72, 95, 115, 123, 145, 149
Herbal Tea(s) 12
Herb(s) 76, 81, 96, 98, 107, 108, 115, 123, 129, 134
Hiatal Hernia 33
Holistic Healing 4
Honey 10, 65, 84, 96, 97, 98, 99, 107, 123, 144
Hops 11
Hormone(s) 8, 9, 28, 68, 89, 107, 112, 121, 133, 145
Hunger 2, 3, 87, 131
Hydrochloric Acid 24, 32, 33, 119
Hydrogenated Fat(s) 69, 73, 144
Hydrogenated Vegetable Oil(s) 9
Hyperactivity 48, 117

I

Ice Cream 25, 65
Immune System 20, 48, 132, 133
Immunity xiv, 5, 20, 139
(Infant) Formula(s) 62, 131, 133
Infectious Diseases 16, 91, 109

EDGAR CAYCE

Edgar Cayce (1877-1945) is known as the world's best-documented psychic, whose legacy includes over 14,000 verbatim transcripts of psychic discourses catalogued in the library of the Association for Research and Enlightenment, Inc., in Virginia Beach, Virginia.

The topics of the Cayce readings, as these discourses are called, range from metaphysical issues and spiritual development to earth-change predictions and medical conditions. More than half of the readings address ~~~~ concerns and provide treatment suggestions ~~~~ orthodox in nature and are based on ~~~~ and remedies. Many of these have ~~~~ tried and tested by medical profes- ~~~~ nical settings. Nutrition is considered ~~~~ nt link in Cayce's holistic approach to

BUSINESS REPLY MAIL

FIRST CLASS   PERMIT NO. 2456   VIRGINIA BEACH, VA

POSTAGE WILL BE PAID BY ADDRESSEE

NO POSTAGE
NECESSARY
IF MAILED
IN THE
UNITED STATES

ASSOCIATION FOR RESEARCH
AND ENLIGHTENMENT INC
215 67TH STREET
VIRGINIA BEACH VA   23451-9819

NATE SAINT

On a Wing and a Prayer

JANET & GEOFF BENGE

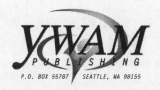

YWAM
PUBLISHING

P.O. BOX 55787   SEATTLE, WA 98155

YWAM Publishing is the publishing ministry of Youth With A Mission (YWAM), an international missionary organization of Christians from many denominations dedicated to presenting Jesus Christ to this generation. To this end, YWAM has focused its efforts in three main areas: (1) training and equipping believers for their part in fulfilling the Great Commission (Matthew 28:19), (2) personal evangelism, and (3) mercy ministry (medical and relief work).

For a free catalog of books and materials, call (425) 771-1153 or (800) 922-2143. Visit us online at www.ywampublishing.com.

Nate Saint: On a Wing and a Prayer
Copyright © 1998 by YWAM Publishing

Published by YWAM Publishing
a ministry of Youth With A Mission
P.O. Box 55787, Seattle, WA 98155-0787

ISBN 978-1-57658-017-2 (paperback)
ISBN 978-1-57658-567-2 (e-book)

Tenth printing 2016

Printed in the United States of America

CHRISTIAN HEROES: THEN & NOW

Available in paperback, e-book, and audiobook formats. Unit study curriculum guides are available for select biographies.

www.HeroesThenAndNow.com

Ecuador

Central Oriente

N

Rio Napo

Shandia

Arajuno   15 minutes by air   Palm Beach

20 minutes by air

5 minutes by air   Rio   Curaray

Auca (Waorani)
settlement
(site of gift drop)

Road from Quito
and Ambato

20 minutes by air

SHELL MERA   Villano   Rio Villano

30 minutes by air

Mt. Sangay

Macuma   Rio   Pastaza

0   10   20 miles

0   ½   1 inch
Scale

This book is dedicated to the Waorani Church elders:

Tementa Nenquihui
Kimo Yeti
Mincayi Enquedi
Yowi Tañi
Kenta Huamoñi
Toñi Toñi

Three of these men participated in the attack at Palm Beach before God transformed their lives. All serve their tribe as evangelists, Bible translators, and Bible teachers. Their faith and hard work have given substance to Nate Saint's hope for the Waorani.

Special thanks to Marj Saint Van Der Puy and Steve Saint for their help in preparing this manuscript.

Contents

Chapter 1

A Whole New World

Nate Saint turned and waited for his nineteen-year-old brother Sam to give him a leg up into the cockpit. He wished he could have swung his leg over himself, but seven-year-old legs just aren't long enough for some things. Sam gave him a good heave, and Nate tumbled into the leather seat. He wiggled around until he was sitting comfortably, then reached for the goggles hanging in front of him. As he sat in the Challenger biplane waiting for Sam to finish his ground check, Nate could hardly believe he was actually going to go flying. In 1930, most adults hadn't been in an airplane, but young Nate had a brother who was a flying instructor.

Finally, Sam climbed into the cockpit behind Nate. Nate heard him flick some switches, and then the engine came to life. The propeller whirled faster and faster in front of Nate until it seemed to disappear. Sam released the brake, and the plane lurched forward. He guided the aircraft to the end of the runway, where he pulled the throttle lever all the way to the "Full" position. The engine screamed louder and louder. The whole plane vibrated in time to its scream as the Challenger began to speed down the runway. Nate could feel his heart pumping fast as the plane skipped off the dirt runway and into the air.

Nate felt cold air rustling through his curly blond hair. He sat up as high as he could in his seat. He craned his neck and tried to see over the side of the plane, but he was just too short. Sam laughed at his effort and then banked the plane slightly to the right. Now Nate could see clearly. They were circling Huntingdon, the town just outside Philadelphia, Pennsylvania, where the Saint family lived. In the distance, Nate could make out the shapes of some of the buildings in downtown Philadelphia. He could also see the two tall, red brick chimneys of the coal-fired power generating plant on the edge of the Delaware River. Nate tried to remember every single minute of the flight so he could tell his friends at school all about it.

When Nate got to school on Monday, the teacher was a little surprised to hear that his parents had allowed him to do something as dangerous as flying.

But then, she didn't know his family. The Saints had a reputation around Huntingdon for being a bit different. In some ways, Nate's parents, Katherine and Lawrence Saint, were very strict parents to their seven sons, Sam, Phil, Dan, David, Steve, Nate, and Ben, and their one daughter, Rachel, especially about religious things. Sunday in the Saint household was the Lord's Day, and after breakfast, the whole family went to Sunday school at the local Presbyterian church. After Sunday school, they would all attend the morning church service and then go home for lunch and family devotions, which included prayer and Bible study. After dinner, they all went off to church for another service. They also went to the weekly Wednesday night prayer meeting at the church. Beside the stove in the kitchen was a big jar of pennies from which they could take a penny for every chapter of the Bible they read to themselves.

For seven years, since Nate had been born, his father had spent nearly all his time in church. He wasn't the pastor; he was much too shy for that. Instead, he was an artist who specialized in reproducing stained-glass windows from the thirteenth century, and he was in charge of making the stained-glass windows for the Washington Cathedral in Washington, D.C. Sometimes he would take Nate and show him his work. And when he did, Nate could look up at the large window in the St. John's chapel and see himself. Yes, see himself. When Nate was five, his father had used him as the model for the stained-glass window of the boy giving Jesus his five loaves and two fishes.

As strict as his parents may have seemed, in other ways they weren't strict at all. A lot of things that bothered most mothers didn't worry Mrs. Saint one bit. Meals at the house were served at all hours of the day and night, whenever enough of the children gathered to make it worth setting the table. The Saints didn't worry if the children didn't eat their vegetables or if they had two desserts and no main course. Nor did they care if the children didn't keep their rooms tidy or had holes in their pants, or even if they were late for school.

Since Mr. Saint was rather forgetful, Nate's mother took care of most of the practical matters around the house. She was organized but, to most people, in a different way. For example, the Saints' three-story wood frame house had a large room with hooks and shelves all around the walls. When all the family's laundry had been ironed, it was placed on the shelves or hung on the hooks. When any of the children needed clean clothes, they went to the room and found something to wear that fit them. It was a case of first up, best dressed! The system gave Mrs. Saint a little spare time to write her poetry and play the piano.

Because her father, Josiah K. Proctor, was an inventor, Mrs. Saint thought it was important to let the children experiment. In the late nineteenth century, he had invented machinery that made woolen mills operate more efficiently. He had started a company called Proctor and Schwartz, which later became Proctor Silex. This had made him a wealthy man. Despite being raised in a wealthy home, Mrs. Saint knew that having ideas and trying new things were more important than having lots of money. It was something she never forgot when she had her own children.

Indeed, more often than not, Mrs. Saint helped the children carry out their wild schemes. When the children came to her with an idea, instead of no, she would say why not? One time when Nate was only four years old, his big brothers Sam and David decided it would be great to sleep on the roof. Their mother thought it was a wonderful idea, too, and she and the children worked out how to make it happen.

Soon the household was buzzing with activity. Mrs. Saint arranged for a carpenter to build a fence around the flat part of the second-story roof over the kitchen. Then she had him build five cots. Extra blankets were found in the attic, and within a week, the family had a new "sleeping room" on the roof. Mrs. Saint and the children all dragged their blankets and pillows out a third-story window and onto the roof. Rachel, who was nine years older than Nate, would read bedtime stories to the younger children by flashlight. Nate remembered the story of David Livingston she read from the book *Fifty Missionary Stories Every Child Should Know*. Somehow, outside on a starry night, the whole adventure seemed more real than ever. For years afterwards, Nate spent many summer nights up in the "roof bedroom."

Of course, Nate's friends loved to spend time at his house. The house was set on an acre of land, and every bit of it was jam-packed with possibilities. Behind the studio where his father did his glass work was the Saint family's private, double-track roller coaster. The huge wooden structure had curves to swoop around and drops to plunge down. Mr. Saint had built it in his spare time with the boys. A few stray nails had gone through the roof of the house and caused leaks, but no one worried too much about that. Nate's parents thought it was more important for the children to have fun and to learn something than to keep everything in perfect condition. Some of the adults in the neighborhood thought the Saints were a little odd, but there was always a line of kids wanting to ride the roller coaster or play in the fifty-foot swing that dangled from the tall elm tree.

Nate and his brothers also loved to make models of anything that moved: trains, boats, airplanes. Nate built a six-foot-long glider from a photo in a book, and he and Philip and Ben made a huge model railroad, which they continued to add to for several years. They called it the B and T and P Depression Railroad, for Ben, Thaney (Nate's nickname), and Philip, and because the country was in the middle of something called the Great Depression. Plus, the words sounded long and important to the boys.

Nate was always getting ideas about how to build things better or stronger. He won prizes at the nearby Abington hobby show for some of his inventions. One of his winning entries was a miniature train he made from scraps of metal left over from one of his father's window frames.

When Nate was ten years old, he got his second airplane ride. Sam landed a shiny, new 1933 Stinson aircraft at a nearby airport. Nate could hardly wait to climb aboard. Best of all, though, this plane had an enclosed cockpit with the seats side by side and two sets of controls. Nate sat down in the right-hand seat and tightened the lap belt as far as it would go. The belt still hung loosely around his small waist. Sam, sitting in the pilot's seat on the left, pulled some levers and flicked several switches. The propeller began to turn and the engine kicked in. The cockpit of the Stinson filled with a powerful hum. Nate watched the needles on the gauges of the instrument panel in front of him and Sam. The needles vibrated gently to the throb of the engine. Sam adjusted some more levers and set the flaps for take-off. He looked around to make sure no one was in the way before releasing the brake lever and touching the throttle to get the engine revving a little faster.

The Stinson aircraft rolled forward. Sam guided the plane all the way to the end of the runway, where he turned it around to face into the wind. Nate watched as Sam pushed the throttle all the way forward. The engine roared, and the Stinson leapt forward. As its wheels pounded up and down on the dirt runway, the plane jerked and twisted. Then the twisting and jerking stopped. Nate looked out the side window of the plane and watched the ground fall away below them. They were airborne.

They flew east across the Delaware River and out over New Jersey. Sam pushed his foot on the right rudder pedal and turned the control wheel. Nate again looked out the side window. He watched as the aileron on the Stinson's wing flicked up and the plane banked toward the south.

After they had been flying awhile, Sam motioned for Nate to take the controls. Sam showed him how to position his feet on the rudder pedals and how to hold the control wheel. Nate had to stretch to get his feet all the way to the pedals, but he made it. Then he put his hands on the wheel. It was amazing. He could feel the throbbing vibration of the engine through the control wheel. He pulled back gently on the wheel, and the nose of the Stinson began to climb. He pushed the wheel forward, and the nose dropped toward the ground below them. It was more thrilling to Nate than riding the roller coaster in the backyard.

A whole new world opened up to Nate that day. From then on, he knew without a doubt that he wanted to be around airplanes for the rest of his life. And everyone around him knew it, too. Airplanes were all he talked about. He drew pictures of airplanes, read about airplanes, and made countless airplane models. And Nate dreamed of the day when he would fly his own plane, just like Sam.

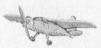

Chapter 2

Nothing Would Stop
Him Now

It was springtime 1937, and fourteen-year-old Nate was stuck in bed. His mind was active, but his body wasn't. His right leg ached so badly he couldn't get out of bed, not even to go to the bathroom. Mrs. Saint liked to give her children vitamins and healthy food to make them better, but when she took Nate's temperature, she called the doctor right away. Something was seriously wrong. Dr. Allen examined Nate's leg. He paid special attention to a small cut Nate received when he had fallen off a sled the week before. Nate was puzzled. The cut was nearly healed, so why was the doctor paying so much attention to it?

After a few minutes, Dr. Allen closed his bag and went downstairs to have a serious talk with

Mrs. Saint. He explained that Nate had osteomyelitis, a bone infection, in his right leg. Bacteria had traveled from the cut on his leg into his bone. Dr. Allen wished there were drugs he could prescribe to help fight the infection, but there were none. All he could do was give Nate some painkillers. The only thing that would help Nate was complete rest. The doctor hoped that with his body at rest, Nate's immune system would fight off the infection. If the infection spread to his knee or ankle, it would lock up, and Nate would be lame for life. But Dr. Allen told Mrs. Saint that even if everything went well and Nate's body fought off the infection, Nate would probably be in bed for months.

The days dragged on. Dr. Allen made many visits, but it was difficult for him to say whether Nate was improving or not. Nate slept a lot, but when he was awake, his family spent as much time as they could keeping him company. Their visits kept his mind off the incredible pain that shot up and down his leg. Nate's older sister, Rachel, spent hours sitting with him and reading him stories. His brothers stopped in to tell him about their latest hunting or fishing trip or to complain about all their homework. Mrs. Saint brought Nate history and art books to read, and Nate's father often stopped in to pray with him.

Still, the Saint household had to go on, and there were many times when Nate lay alone in bed. He would think back to the summer before, when he had been at camp in the Poconoes. He especially liked to think about the Saturday night when they were all seated around the campfire. The counselor had asked who wanted to invite Jesus into their life. Nate had raised his hand. All his life he had heard Bible stories and said his prayers, but that night it all became real to him. It was the difference between seeing his father's pencil sketch of a magnificent stained-glass window and seeing the light glow through the real, finished window itself.

As he lay alone in his room, Nate spent a lot of time reading his Bible and praying. He knew his infection was serious and that he could possibly die from it. While that knowledge didn't really frighten him, he realized he was young and had so much life ahead of him. So he prayed and promised God that if he lived, he would turn his whole life over to God.

Finally, after several weeks, Dr. Allen announced that Nate was beginning to heal. Nate's body had fought off the infection, and the pain in his leg began to diminish. Nate started feeling a lot better, and before long he was restless and looking for projects he could do from his bed. He drew plans for a sailboat he wanted to build. He designed the boat with a rounded hull, unlike any other sailboat he'd ever seen. Somehow he knew the design would make the boat sail well. He also made papier-mache models. The hours sped by as he ripped up newspaper, pasted it, and molded it into shape. When the models dried, he painted them. He made a huge mask using this same process and had lots of fun scaring people who came to visit him.

As he got better, Nate wanted to spend more time downstairs in the living room. Since his leg was still too painful to walk on, the family got used to him crawling around the house on his hands and knees.

By the time Nate was finally better, he had a lot of schoolwork to catch up on. But he also didn't forget the promise he'd made to God. He kept up his prayer and Bible study and became president of the Baptist Young People's Union. He also taught junior Sunday school at Bethany Baptist Church, where the family now attended.

Nate also pulled out the plans he'd drawn while he was sick. It was time to build the sailboat. This time he wasn't building a model, but a full-sized boat. He had designed the boat to be eight feet long and nearly as wide. It looked like half a ball with a mast and sail stuck in the middle. When he showed his brothers the plans, they just laughed and told him a boat that shape might float, but it would never go fast. Nate ignored them, smiled, and began building the boat.

Of course, making a boat from scratch is a difficult job, but Nate enjoyed overcoming each new problem the construction faced him with. He had to figure out how to get the planks on the outside of the hull to bend without breaking. He experimented until he discovered that wet wood can be molded without breaking. He worked out how long he needed to soak the mahogany planks before he could form them into the curved shape of the hull.

He spent hours sewing the sails on his mother's treadle sewing machine and made all the metal fittings for the boat, as well. Finally, the boat was finished, and Nate proudly painted the name *Sinbad* on its bow and the home port of *Bagdad* on its stern.

He sailed *Sinbad* on the Delaware River. She skimmed upriver, leaving bigger, more expensive boats in her wake. Nate gripped the tiller and grinned at his brother David, who was manning the mainsail. His design worked even better than he'd thought it would. Somehow as the wind filled the sails, the tiny boat lifted in the water and skimmed effortlessly and speedily across the surface. Nate felt completely satisfied as he guided *Sinbad* up the river. Nothing made him happier than to plan something, make it, and then use it.

Whenever he had to sit for a long time, Nate became restless. He wanted to be out doing something, not sitting around. Because of this, school tested him, and by his senior year in high school, he was ready for something else. He tried working at night and going to school during the day, but that tired him out. So he reversed the order. He dropped out of day school and went to night school in Philadelphia while he worked during the day in a welding and machine shop. That suited Nate much better; he was doing things with his hands and using his brain at the same time.

Nate graduated from high school in 1941. As he graduated, the world was changing. World War II had been going on for nearly two years in Europe and Asia, and there were rumors that the United States was going to get involved in the war. Such rumors made it hard for a young man to concentrate on a career, so Nate drifted from job to job. He started working in a welding and machine shop and then switched to tree trimming. Then he tried pumping gas at a local gas station. All the while, Nate felt restless. He hadn't found his niche, and it was hard for him to focus long on any one thing.

Nate thought he'd like to travel, so he agreed to deliver a truck to a missionary family in the hills of southwest Virginia. However, things didn't work out as smoothly as he thought they would. Once he'd delivered the truck, he had no way to get home. He decided to hitchhike. There was just one problem: There weren't many vehicles on the back roads of Virginia, so getting a ride wasn't easy. As Nate stood by the side of a road waiting for a car headed north to come by, he noticed a train in the distance. The railroad track ran along close to the road and then took a sharp bend to the north. *Surely the train has to slow down for the bend*, Nate thought to himself. He ran over to the bend in the tracks and waited for the train to get closer. As it approached, it slowed, and Nate began running alongside. When a boxcar came by with its doors open, he effortlessly swung his body through the door and into the empty boxcar.

Nate sat by the door congratulating himself on how easy it had been to hitch a ride on a freight train. As he looked around the dim interior of the empty boxcar, he noticed several dark shapes. As his eyes adjusted to the faint light, the shapes turned into hobos, homeless men who rode the trains from one part of the country to another in search of jobs or food. Nate was surprised by them at first, but he and the men got along fine.

Nate was thoroughly enjoying his free ride until the train stopped in Bluefield, Virginia. The Bluefield police regularly searched for hobos on the trains passing through town. Nate surely didn't look like a hobo, but he was on a train without a ticket, and as he soon found out, that was illegal.

The hobos and Nate were taken before a judge. They all stood in a line in the courtroom. The judge looked at each of them sternly and pronounced his sentence: a ten-dollar fine and ten days in the local jail. When the judge got to Nate, he hesitated and took another look. Anyone could see Nate was not a hobo, so the judge pointed at him and said, "Your sentence, son, is ten dollars *or* ten days in jail. One or the other. Which will it be?"

Nate knew the judge was being kind and trying to spare him from having to go to jail, but Nate had more time than money. "I'll take the jail time, Your Honor," he replied. And with that he went to jail for the one and only time in his life.

Nate sent three postcards from his jail cell back to Huntingdon. On the first he complained the potatoes were so hard he could bounce them off the floor. On the second he drew a sketch of an escape plan, and on the third he wrote in huge letters the word *FREE*. After his release, Nate hitchhiked home from Bluefield, keeping a safe distance from freight trains.

Whatever Nate was doing, his thoughts were never far from airplanes. In mid-1941 he got a job at an airfield on the outskirts of Philadelphia as a general hand for the Flying Dutchman Air Service, where big brother Sam had worked as a flight instructor. He was around airplanes, and he began to feel his life was on track again. On June 16, 1941, while working at the airfield, Nate took his first official flying lesson. From then on, he saved every penny until he was able to buy himself a small airplane in which he could build up his flying hours, and eventually he got his private pilot's license.

Meanwhile, Sam had become a pilot for American Airlines, and he arranged for Nate to become an apprentice aircraft mechanic for the airline at La Guardia Field in New York City. It was an exciting time for Nate, who moved to New York and stayed with Sam, Sam's wife Jeanne, and their four-year-old daughter.

On December 7,1941, while Nate was working in New York, the biggest news story since the start of the Great Depression broke. Japan had attacked the United States at Pearl Harbor in Hawaii. It all seemed so far away as Nate read about the attack in the *New York Times*. When the United States in response declared war on Japan and began drafting men and women into the armed services, it didn't affect Nate. The airline industry was an "essential industry," which meant that people like Nate and Sam who worked for airlines could not be drafted into the military, because their jobs were too important. So, as the United States entered World War II, Nate kept right on working as an apprentice airplane mechanic, knowing he would not be drafted.

But as 1942 rolled on, Nate became restless. All around him married men, many with young children, were being called up to go overseas to fight in very dangerous situations. Yet here he was, a single man with a "safe" job. Something about the situation bothered him. It didn't seem fair. Of course, there was one simple solution, but it was not a solution that would make him popular with his boss.

Finally, just before Thanksgiving, Nate got up the courage to tell his boss he was going to quit his apprenticeship and sign up for the Army Air Corps. His boss was very unhappy. Nate was a good worker, and his boss could not understand why someone would leave a "safe" job that thousands of other men would gladly take. But Nate stood firm. He was ready to go wherever his country sent him.

He made several trips to Washington, D.C., to apply for the Army Air Corps, but in the end he was accepted into the regular army. To get in, he had to take a six-hour physical exam, during which the doctors found the scars from his osteomyelitis. They were concerned that he'd had such a serious illness, but in the end he passed the exam. The doctors wrote a note in his records that read, "Accepted for Limited Service." Nate was so glad to pass the medical examination that he didn't give the note in his record a second thought. He certainly couldn't have imagined the impact it would have on his life in the years to come.

Nate spent Christmas 1942 at home in Huntingdon Valley with family and friends. Then, on December 30, he took a train back to New York to join the army. From New York he was shipped off to Camp Luna in Las Vegas, New Mexico. Nate thought it would be nice and warm out there, but a surprise awaited him when he arrived. Camp Luna was located in the Sangre Mountains, and any thoughts of balmy nights and a suntan quickly faded as he trudged through three inches of snow to get to his tent.

Nate had joined the army to learn new skills, like flying commercial airplanes, but his first job involved using a skill he'd learned years ago at home in Huntingdon: cleaning toilets! Still, someone had to do it, and Nate did it with the same enthusiasm he showed when fixing an airplane.

Life quickly fell into a routine at Cape Luna. Nate was up at five in the morning for parade and barracks inspection. Then there was breakfast before the troops were marched out to learn all the skills necessary for fighting a war. They did fitness training and learned survival skills. By lights-out, Nate would fall into bed exhausted, but he was always up the next morning ready to go.

Whenever he got the chance, Nate went into town to church. News soon spread that he was a

Christian, and other Christians sought him out to pray with them. Nate also arranged Bible studies for other Christians in his unit.

All the while, Nate never gave up on his dream of flying, even though he knew it wasn't easy to get flying jobs in the U.S. Army. Still, his persistence paid off, and he was accepted into a training program in Los Angeles. In the program he would learn to work on the C-47 cargo planes that the military used to transport men and supplies. At the training school, Nate studied in class from two in the afternoon until one o'clock in the morning. He learned all he could, and after graduating from the training program in March 1943, he was sent to an Army base in the Mojave Desert to work on C-47s. From there he was sent to Jefferson Barracks, St. Louis, Missouri.

All this moving around got a little tiresome. Nate had been in the army for only four months, and already he'd been from New York to New Mexico to California and now to Missouri. Sometimes he felt like he barely had time to unpack all his things before he got his orders to move on to his next assignment. He figured that if he kept that pace up, he could well see the entire United States at Uncle Sam's expense. But as much as he liked to see new places and new things, bouncing around from one place to another had its share of problems. Mail, for example, usually took a while to catch up to him. Sometimes letters went to two or three places before he received them.

Jefferson Barracks was a crossroad for many soldiers who were shipped in to learn important things about fighting in a war and then were shipped out all over the world to fight for the United States.

Nate enjoyed learning new things, especially if it was hands-on and not just from a book. In St. Louis, he learned how to survive a gas attack and use a variety of weapons safely. While he didn't like the idea of ever using a gun in a real battle, he enjoyed learning how guns worked. Once the soldiers understood how the various guns and rifles worked, they were expected to be able to take them completely apart and put them back together again without help or instruction manuals. Nate went one step further: He practiced until he could strip the guns down and put them back together in the dark! It wasn't difficult for a kid who'd been pulling his mother's appliances and clocks apart since he was a small boy.

Finally, after several months at Jefferson Barracks, Nate got the letter he'd been waiting for since enlisting in the army. The letter was addressed to "Saint, Nathaniel. 28th Training Group." Nate's hands trembled as he opened it. He took a deep breath before unfolding the letter. To his delight, the letter read, "You have been accepted into the Air Cadet Training Program. Please report to Morningside College, Sioux City, Iowa, at 2100 hours on June 12, 1943."

"Yippee!" Nate let out in a yell of excitement that brought his friends to see what was up. He showed them the letter. Finally, he was going to get to fly for the U.S. Army!

Nate hardly had time to pack his things and write to his parents before he was on his way to Sioux City, Iowa. As the train chugged along, he sat with fifty other cadets, but his thoughts were far away. He thought back to his first flight with Sam. It had been so exciting to feel the wind rustle through his hair and whistle around his ears. And it felt like electricity running through his body when Sam banked the plane and Nate looked down on the Delaware River from three thousand feet up. Now, thirteen years later, he was on his way to become an Army pilot. His dream was about to come true. He felt that same electricity in his body. Nothing would stop him now.

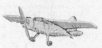

Chapter 3

A Different Kodachrome Slide

H up two, hup two, hup two." Nate marched along to the rhythmic chant of the drill sergeant. He had been at Morningside College in Sioux City for three months now. The routine was tough but bearable. There were endless lectures and tests, fitness exercises, duties, and drills like the night march he was on. But it was all worth it, and now he was only two days away from beginning the best part of all: flight training.

As he marched in time with the other cadets across the darkened parade ground and around behind the mess hall, Nate thought of all the possibilities that lay ahead of him. The war was going strong; American and English troops had invaded and captured Sicily, and now they were preparing for an invasion of Italy. In the Pacific, American troops were forcing the Japanese back island by island. Many people thought there was a good chance the war would be over before long. Nate wondered if he might not even get to experience active duty. But even if he didn't, he knew his training would land him a good job as a commercial pilot. Perhaps Sam might be able to help him get into American Airlines. How exciting that would be; instead of greasing and fueling the planes, he would be piloting them.

By now, all the cadets were lined up behind the mess hall for a final inspection before being dismissed for supper. As usual, the food was terrible. Nate often joked that if the army served up dirty dishwater, most of the soldiers would have a hard time recognizing that it wasn't soup. Still, he was hungry, and he ate what he needed before heading for bed and a good night's sleep.

His roommate, Bob Bjorklund, was already in bed when he got to the room. Nate wished him goodnight and sat on the edge of his cot. He pulled off his boots, and then his socks. He didn't know exactly why his right leg felt a little sore. He figured he must have bumped it during the march. Standing up, he pulled off his trousers, and as he did, his heart fell. The impossible had happened. There was a red swelling around the old osteomyelitis scar on his leg. It could mean only one thing: the infection was back.

Without saying a word to Bob, Nate took off the rest of his clothes and got into bed. He pulled the blanket tight around his body, hoping that in some magical way it would keep out not only the cold but also his thoughts. In the dark of the night, though, the thoughts seeped into his head. He didn't need a doctor to tell him that his flying days were over before they had begun. Hot tears welled up in his eyes and slid silently across his cheeks and onto the pillow. Years of anticipation drained out of him with the tears. It was over, all over. The next morning Nate did what he knew he had to do. He reported to the base doctor, who told him what he already knew—the osteomyelitis was back.

The following day was his twentieth birthday, but instead of going to the airport for his first day of flying with the other cadets, he bid them farewell from outside his barracks. He took a snapshot of them all smiling in anticipation of the flying that lay ahead. Then Nate climbed into an Army jeep and was taken to the hospital for x-rays. It was a birthday he did not want to remember, but one he knew he would never forget.

He wrote a letter to his parents and told them the disappointing news. He wrote: "The way the situation has changed during the last couple of days reminds me of that dog in Bryn Athyn that used to chase me when I rode past with my newspapers. I remember how he put it in reverse the day I dropped a firecracker in front of him. He skidded about ten feet forward while running backward before he stopped....I've just stopped—which direction I'll take off, I don't know."

He folded the letter and enclosed the snapshot of the other cadets on their way to the airport. He marked a little "x" where he would have been positioned if he'd been with them. But he wasn't with them, and there was nothing he could do about it. Life would have to go on. Despite his disappointment, somewhere deep inside he knew God had things under control, and in God he would trust.

The x-rays confirmed that Nate's osteomyelitis had indeed flared up again. It quickly settled down again, too, but a man with a medical problem could not be considered for duty overseas. The doctor stamped "Disqualified for Combat Crew Duty" on his record, and that was the end of the matter. The army would never train him to fly now if he couldn't go into combat in an airplane.

For the next month, Nate was assigned to non-flying duties. Without the pressure of study or preparing to fly, he had a lot of time on his hands. He spent much of it reading and praying. One magazine he liked to read was *Reader's Digest*, and in the August 1943 issue he read about a new "wonder drug" called penicillin, which reportedly was able to stop infections. Nate thought of his osteomyelitis and that it was too bad penicillin hadn't been discovered ten years earlier when he first needed it.

After a month, Nate was transferred yet again, this time to Amarillo, Texas, where he was made the barracks chief in charge of fifty men. It turned out to be a lot harder work than he'd imagined, getting fifty men up and inspected each morning, but he enjoyed the challenge. Nate found a group of Christian men in the barracks and developed friendships with them. He also inspired several other soldiers to renew their commitment to God.

Again, with the pressure of study off, Nate had plenty of spare time, and the Army base at Amarillo seemed to Nate to be the most boring place on earth. Nate needed something to keep him busy and take his mind off not being an army pilot. Thankfully, one of the other soldiers introduced him to the base's photography department, which had a large darkroom and camera equipment available for soldiers to use free of charge. Nate took to photography. He loved both the artistic side of it— getting just the right light and the right camera angle for a shot—and the practical side, mixing chemicals and developing his film and photographs in the darkroom. Nate's favorite subjects to photograph were people going about their daily routines. He made photos of enlisted men polishing their boots, sergeants driving jeeps, cooks mixing biscuits. No one on base escaped the attention of Nate Saint and his camera.

Nate also used his spare time to write long, interesting letters. It was hard for him to believe a year had gone by since he'd signed up in New York. Now he was about to spend his first Christmas away from home. In a letter to his parents written just before Christmas 1943, he said: "Two fellows just closed the barracks door, leaving me alone....They left a radio on and I can hear distantly, 'O Come Let

Us Adore Him.' There's snow on the ground and the stars are glittering clearly—like gems on black velvet, illuminated by a great hidden light...." He went on in the letter to tell how he was about to be transferred yet again. "They have made up special orders for me to proceed to Fort Wayne, Indiana. If flying is 'out,' I want to be useful in some way. It will feel good to get greasy, get a few callouses, skin my knuckles on a gadget, hurry to get 'er ready to go on time, and go to bed really tired again."

Once again, Nate settled into a new routine, this time at Baer Field in Fort Wayne. He was a crew chief working on C-47 transport aircraft. It was an interesting job, but just as in Amarillo, he had a lot of spare time.

One of the soldiers he worked with had just qualified for his license as a class E airplane mechanic. Until then, Nate had not been aware that the army would help mechanics become better qualified for other positions. It was an opportunity too good to miss, so Nate, who had left his apprenticeship at American Airlines early, now threw himself into studying for his class E aircraft mechanic's license.

When he needed a break from study, he would drive over to the Winona Lake Bible Conference grounds about forty miles east of Fort Wayne. Nate's older brother Phillip, who had become a well-known artist and evangelist, often spoke there. The two brothers spent many happy evenings talking together around the campfire. It was just like old times on the roof back in Huntingdon.

From time to time, Nate was sent from Baer Field on special assignments. In early November 1944, he was sent for several weeks to the Willow Run plant of the Ford Motor Company near Detroit. The plant was producing a new type of airplane engine, and because of his mechanical ability, Nate was asked to investigate the engine and report to the engineers back at Baer Field. Nate found the assignment interesting, but something else happened on the trip that totally changed his life.

For some time, Nate had been listening to Dr. John Zoller's radio broadcasts. Since he was so close to Detroit, it seemed like a good opportunity to visit Dr. Zoller's church and hear him speak in person. And so on New Year's Eve in 1944, Nate made his way to the Zoller Gospel Tabernacle in Detroit. He went into the church service with an ambition to be a pilot or an aircraft mechanic in the United States, but when he came out of the church in the early hours of New Year's Day, 1945, he had decided to go to Bible school and then become a missionary in some foreign country.

He wrote about this transformation in a letter home: "Now, you've heard people tell about God speaking to them, haven't you? I don't know about the other fellow, but that night I saw things differently...BING...like that. Just as though a different Kodachrome slide had been tossed onto the screen between my ears."

That night Nate realized how much time and effort he'd wasted going after his own dreams and plans, and he understood the deep joy that comes from surrendering every dream and plan and talent back to God. As this understanding grew in his mind during the church service, Nate decided to give up his dreams of flying commercially and enroll in a Bible college once the war was over. He wrote in his diary soon after the service: "The Lord has given me no desire to preach, but I'd like someday to be able to tell somebody who has never heard...."

After six weeks at the Ford plant, Nate returned to Baer Field. When he got back, he recognized his father's handwriting on the envelope of a letter from home. He ripped it open. His father didn't normally write, so Nate was eager to know what he had to say. Inside the envelope was a brief note from Mr. Saint and an article he'd cut from the *Sunday School Times.* The article, entitled "On Wings of the Wind," was written by a navy pilot, Jim Truxton. The article described a new organization that Truxton and an ex-Air Force WASP pilot, Betty Greene, had just founded.

Nate read on. The organization was called Christian Airmen's Missionary Fellowship, or CAMF for short. CAMF had been formed to serve missionaries who were working in remote areas of the world by flying in supplies for them, carrying the supplies to a doctor when the missionaries needed medical help, and ferrying them quickly from place to place. Although the new organization did not yet have an airplane, the article invited airmen who were interested in the new ministry to reply to their Los Angeles office.

Nate sat on his cot and read the article through several times. He didn't know what to think. He had just given up the idea of flying and had dedicated himself to becoming a missionary. But now, while reading the article, Nate was starting to realize that God might be showing him a way to be a missionary *and* fly. He thought about it. He had both an aircraft mechanic's license and a private pilot's license, two qualifications CAMF was looking for. He decided to write a letter to Jim Truxton.

Nate started the letter by saying: "Last New Year's Eve in a watch-night service I responded to the missionary challenge. [I] have been interested in missionary work for some time but the Lord owned only my finances. He now has my life." Nate went on to list his educational background and qualifications, and then he folded the letter and slipped it into an envelope. As he dropped the letter into the mailbox at Baer Field, he had no idea it would lead to the greatest adventures of his life.

Chapter 4

An Unacceptable Risk

Nate received a fast reply from Christian Airmen's Missionary Fellowship. Betty Greene wrote about CAMF's plans to begin work in South America. CAMF's first goal was to help Wycliffe Bible Translators set up some jungle stations in southern Mexico and then do the same in Peru. Betty Greene suggested that when the war was over, Nate join her in Peru and become the ministry's mechanic. Nate thought and prayed long and hard about her offer.

Meanwhile, army life continued as usual. There were new challenges and new locations. For a while, Nate briefed crews going into combat overseas. He loved the job; it gave him regular hours and an office of his own. Best of all, though, he got

49

Sundays off. And every Sunday, Nate would be in
church, usually with a few fellow soldiers he'd
brought along with him.

On June 19, 1945, after eighteen months stationed at Baer Field, Nate was transferred to an air
base near Salinas, California. Shortly afterwards, he
was transferred yet again, this time to Castle Field
in Merced, California. Soon after Nate arrived in
Merced, in August, the Japanese surrendered to the
United States. World War II was over, the war effort
began to wind down, and everyone stationed at the
base had more time on their hands. Nate used the
extra time to tell others about the gospel message.
He invited friends to church with him and began
holding a regular Bible study on the base. As a
result of the Bible study and the example of his life,
many men became committed Christians.

While stationed at Merced, Nate continued to
think and pray about the offer from Betty Greene.
In the end, though, he felt he should go to Bible college first and get some theological training.
Reluctantly, he wrote to Betty Greene and turned
down her offer—for now.

About this time, Nate was also thinking about
Marjorie Farris, a friend of a friend. Marj, as she
liked to be called, was training to be a nurse in Los
Angeles. She was about five-foot-two with short,
wavy brown hair and sparkling blue eyes. Nate had
met her only a few times, but there was something
about her faith and the way she cared for those
around her that attracted him. Marj lived in a flurry

of activity, always visiting friends, volunteering her spare time to sit with ill patients, and leading Sunday school at a local church. Despite all her activity, there was a peace about Marj. She was never in a hurry and somehow always had enough time to make everyone she met feel special. Nate would have liked to spend more time with her, but Merced was three hundred miles from Los Angeles, and he expected to be sent home soon to Huntingdon, Pennsylvania, for good.

Men were being discharged from the army and shipped home every week from Castle Field. Nate waited impatiently for his discharge papers to arrive. After nearly three years in the army, he was tired of the routine of military life and the lack of privacy that came with it. As he waited, he came up with the idea of using his remaining leave time to go camping at Yosemite National Park. There he could get away from everything and be alone with nature. Nate had no idea just how alone he would end up being.

Nate set out for Yosemite with two army buddies. It was mid-December, and when they arrived, the park was nearly empty. The following morning, as the three men looked out the tent door, they knew why the park was deserted. It was not normal camping weather. Thick, damp fog had closed in all around them, blanketing them in gray silence. It was hardly the start to the trip they'd imagined, but Nate was eager to do something. He wanted to hike the trail up to Glacier Point. The trail was several miles long, and neither of his two friends was eager to hike it with him. So Nate, determined to do something different on this vacation, decided he'd hike the trail alone.

An hour later, wearing his army issue coveralls with two sweaters pulled over them and carrying a pocketful of peanuts to snack on, he headed up the mountain trail. He waved a cheerful farewell to his buddies and rounded the bend that officially marked the start of the well-used path. Hundreds of people used the trail in the summer, so he thought it wouldn't be too difficult to climb, even in the damp fog. And it would be good to get away from everyone and be able to make his own decisions for once.

Just beyond the trail head, Nate stopped to talk to a park ranger. He told the ranger where he was headed, and the ranger pointed out that it was not the best weather for climbing the mountain. Nate insisted he would be fine. The ranger told him if he got to the top, he would be welcome at the lodge at the end of the trail. Douglas Whiteside, a photographer, was spending the winter there and would love someone to chat with over hot coffee.

Nate could hardy wait to get moving. There was someone to talk to about photography at the end of the trail. He munched a few peanuts as he started up the mountain. There were no forks in the path, and every turn was well marked, so the trail was easy to follow. He whistled as he walked along, happy that there was probably not another person between him and Douglas Whiteside. He hoped, though, that he'd soon climb above the low clouds and drizzle and feel the warmth of the sun on his face. But instead of getting above the low clouds, he entered more and more fog the higher he went. Still, he didn't think too much about it; he was on a well-defined trail, and he could always turn back if conditions got too bad. Besides, a single telephone wire was strung above the trail, and he felt sure it led right to the lodge where Douglas Whiteside was staying.

It wasn't long before the misty drizzle turned to a steady rain. But Nate still didn't worry. He had on two sweaters and a woolen undershirt that kept out the rain. After he had been walking for a while, his muscles began to ache a little, so he walked backwards for a few minutes at a time to stretch them out. Upward he went, one army boot after the other.

As he got higher up the trail, the rain turned to light snow, and before long the light snow gave way to heavy snow. Now Nate was beginning to worry. He had no idea how far it was to the lodge at the top, but the telephone wire was still running along overhead. As Nate walked on, he began making emergency plans in his mind. If he got too exhausted to go any farther, he could break the wire. When the rangers came up to fix the problem, they would find him. Trouble was, if Nate had been thinking more clearly, he would have realized that the wire often broke in winter under the strain of snow and ice or because of landslides. As a result, the rangers usually waited until spring before they would fix the broken wire.

Nate trudged on. It was too late to go back, and he felt sure the lodge couldn't be far away now. The snow was already six inches deep, and it took all his effort to keep one foot moving in front of the other. After a while he had to use his hands to help lift his legs with each step. He was shivering so hard now it was difficult to reach into his pocket for the peanuts, and after putting the peanuts in his mouth, it took all his effort to chew and swallow them. He had to stop every few minutes and rest. He would scoop up a handful of snow and stuff it into his mouth. As his body heat melted it, cold water trickled down the back of his throat. He looked around at the swirling whiteness that surrounded him and smiled to himself. *One thing's for sure,* he thought, *I'll never die of thirst up here.*

He continued to walk, keeping his head down, concentrating on the trail. He could still make out the outline of the trail beneath the snow. He also kept a close lookout for signs of life.

His feet were now damp and cold, and he was having a difficult time feeling his toes. It was also becoming difficult to concentrate on the path in front of him. He was just about to flop down onto the snow from exhaustion when he noticed something. He could hardly believe what he was seeing. He rubbed his eyes and looked again. He wasn't seeing things; there really were footprints in the middle of the trail, and fresh footprints at that! They could only be Douglas Whiteside's footprints. The lodge had to be close by. Footprint by footprint, Nate placed his feet where Whiteside's feet must have trod no more than five minutes before. If it had been any longer than that, the snow would have covered the footprints over.

As Nate trudged on, footprint after footprint, his mind began to tell him there was something strange about what he was doing. But what was it? He was so cold he was having trouble thinking straight. And then it dawned on him. It was the shape of the prints. Douglas Whiteside would be wearing boots in weather like this, but the footprints Nate was following were bootless. Not only that, but the feet making the footprints were each about seven inches wide. Nate fell to his knees and looked closer. The footprints he was following had been made by a huge bear. He had been following a bear up the mountain!

There wasn't much he could do about it now. If there was a bear on the trail ahead of him, he'd just have to deal with the situation when he got to it. Right now it was taking all his effort just to keep moving. He struggled on for about another hundred yards before the bear prints finally left the trail and headed toward a rocky ridge.

Totally exhausted, Nate fell into the snow. His legs would no longer do what his brain told them to do. He felt sure he was going to die right there in the middle of the trail. He didn't fear dying. Instead

he felt angry, angry at himself for getting into the
trouble he was in. How could he have been so
stupid, so careless? He thought back to the New
Year's Eve service in Detroit where he had dedicated himself to be a missionary. Now, because of
his foolishness, he would never realize that dream.
Instead, he had thrown his life away in a foolhardy
hike up a mountain in bad weather.

Sitting there thinking about the trouble he was
in got Nate so angry with himself that somehow he
found the energy to get back on his feet and keep
trudging. As he walked, he began doing something
he should have done a lot earlier: He began to pray.
He didn't plead with God or make any bargains
like, "If you just get me out of this mess, God, I'll do
so and so." No, Nate had already committed his life
to serve God as a missionary after he got out of the
army. Instead, Nate thanked God for all the wonderful things He had done for him. As he prayed
prayers of gratitude, a great feeling of peace came
over him. In fact, he felt happy, and a broad smile
spread across his face.

After a while though, despite the peace he felt
inside, he became so exhausted that his mind went
blank. Somehow his body kept moving. He became
aware of dark shadows ahead of him. As he stum-
bled forward, the shadows became trees. He
searched the sky above him for the phone wire.
Finally, he spotted it running into the trees. With his
eyes now fixed on the wire, he kept on going.
Finally, the wire disappeared into a cabin. He'd

made it! Or had he? There was still another hundred yards to go to reach the cabin, and his body was too exhausted to go on. His legs buckled beneath him, and he slumped face down into the snow. His face was so numb he couldn't even feel the icy cold of the snow pressed against it. *What a shame to walk so far and die within sight of help.* The thought slowly crept across Nate's mind. After several minutes lying in the snow, he again found the energy to will his body to stand up and lurch forward. Stumbling footstep after footstep, he got closer and closer to the lodge. But before he reached the building, he had to stop twice more to gather his energy. At last, he fell against the door of the lodge. He called out. It was a pitiful, breathless call, but somehow it got Douglas Whiteside's attention. As the photographer swung the door open, warm air rushed against Nate's face. Nate pushed past Whiteside and collapsed onto the nearest chair.

Douglas Whiteside was surprised at his unexpected guest, but he quickly sized up the situation. He poured some soup into a pan on the stove and dragged Nate to his bed and took off his wet clothes. Within an hour, Nate was fast asleep with hot soup warming his insides and a well-stoked fire heating his outsides.

The next day Nate told Douglas Whiteside all about his foolish trip. He wanted to head right back down the mountain, but Whiteside suggested he stay put for a while and get his strength back. This time, Nate took the advice.

The following day, Douglas Whiteside walked down the trail with Nate. He made sure they were safely below the snow line before letting Nate walk the last few miles to the start of the trail alone. Nate had left his army buddies two days earlier, excited to be alone for a while. When he got back, he was very glad to see them again. He didn't even think about his lack of privacy as the three of them piled into their tent for the night. In fact, it was quite comforting to hear his buddies snoring away on either side of him.

Nate pulled his sleeping bag around his shoulders and thought about the perilous trip up the mountain. How close he'd come to dying from cold and exposure! And it had happened because he'd been foolhardy. He had taken an unacceptable risk.

He thought about flying. It was risky, too. But it was an acceptable risk, like hiking the trail up to Glacier Point on a warm summer's day would be. In summer, the chances were good that you'd get all the way up there and back safely. If you took some precautions, packed some extra clothes and food, you could minimize the risk even more. Flying was like that. When you took off, there was a good chance you'd land safely. And if you were careful, thoroughly carried out your preflight safety checks, and were sure of where you were headed, you minimized your risk of crashing. But if you were foolhardy and took unacceptable risks, like flying in bad weather or neglecting safety and maintenance checks or making reckless maneuvers, you increased your chances of crashing.

Seeing how close he'd come to throwing his life away because he had taken an unacceptable risk, Nate decided there and then that for the rest of his life he would strive to minimize the risk in the things he did, especially when he was flying. He would never again be foolhardy and ignore the advice of people who clearly knew better than he did about things. With that thought fixed firmly in his mind, Nate fell sound asleep.

Chapter 5

Baskets of Wings

Finally, in February 1946, Nate was formally discharged from the army. It was time for him to head home to Huntingdon. He boarded a long train carrying discharged soldiers back east. At the same time as Nate was winding his way across the country by train, Betty Greene was flying CAMF's first plane to Mexico. It was a four-seater, 220-horsepower, enclosed-cabin Waco biplane.

Once back in Huntingdon, Nate had time on his hands again. He wasn't due to start at Wheaton College until the fall. To fill in the time, he bought himself a secondhand airplane and began using it to build up his flying hours. Before long, he had qualified for his commercial pilot's and instructor's ratings.

Three months after Nate got back home to Huntingdon, an air crash occurred that would change his life, not because he was in it but because he would have to repair the damaged plane. Betty Greene was about to finish her time in Mexico and head for Peru, and George Wiggins, an ex-navy pilot, had come to replace her. They had taken a flight together to familiarize Wiggins with the area and were attempting to land on a tiny airstrip at El Real, about a mile from the Wycliffe Bible Translator's jungle camp in southern Mexico, when their landing went wrong. Fortunately, both pilots had climbed out of the cockpit unhurt, which was more than could be said for the plane, which lay on its side, its two left wings torn off, its propeller bent out of shape, and its landing gear broken.

Betty Greene was aware that the accident could shut down CAMF altogether. Many people were watching the organization to see whether it really was worthwhile and safe to run an airline just for missionaries. As she looked at the wreckage of the Waco biplane, she knew something had to be done fast. She and George Wiggins were both pilots, but neither of them had any idea how to fix a badly damaged airplane in the middle of a tropical jungle. But Betty Greene knew someone who did.

By the time the request for help reached Nate Saint, via Jim Truxton, the details were a little vague. Somewhere in Mexico was a CAMF plane that needed "a bit" of help. After praying about it, Nate decided to put off going to college and give his time to where it was needed most. He called Jim Truxton and told him that, if he was needed, he could be ready to go in as little as two weeks.

Two days later, a letter arrived containing a rail ticket to the Mexican border. The ticket was dated for three days away! Nate raced into action. There was so much to do: photographs to be taken for a passport, visas to be obtained, certified duplicates of his aviation certificates and ratings to be made, his plane to be sold, and a million other little things to be taken care of before he left. Amazingly, on the third day, he was sitting on a train headed south with forty pounds of tools neatly arranged in a tool-box inside his duffel bag. He never let the bag out of his sight. Without his tools, nothing would be getting repaired in Mexico.

The train had crossed the Missouri River into Kansas before it began to dawn on Nate that he'd been too busy getting ready to actually think much about where he was going. He was on a train headed for Laredo on the Texas/Mexico border. But he had not had enough time to study where he should go once he crossed the border. He pulled out the letter Jim Truxton had sent him and read it carefully. The letter contained an apartment address, Apartado 8673, Tuxtla Gtz. Mexico. He had no clue where that was, only that somewhere in Mexico, in an apartment in a place called Gtz., someone was waiting for him!

Then, of course, there was the language barrier. Nate knew that Spanish was spoken in Mexico, but he didn't speak Spanish. As the golden wheat fields of Kansas flashed past his window, marking the journey south, he began to wonder what he'd actually let himself in for. Perhaps once he found the plane, things would be easier. After all, it couldn't be too badly damaged, because they'd asked for only one mechanic to come fix it. Perhaps he could have it flying again and be back home in time for the fall semester of college after all.

The train continued south, and Nate was glad when, on the last day of his trip to the border, four young Mexican men climbed into his carriage. He listened to their Spanish and wondered if he could ever learn to speak the language like they did. In the end, he thought it would take him quite a while to learn to speak it that well, so he had the four young men teach him one phrase in Spanish: "Is there someone here who speaks English?" It seemed the only sensible thing to learn to say. Nate shared with the men the apartment address he was headed for. They looked at it and burst out laughing. It was a long time before they finally settled down enough to tell him that an *apartado* was not an apartment but a post office box. *Great*, thought Nate, *now I'm meeting someone in a post office box in Mexico!*

Together they tackled the job of finding Tuxtla Gtz. on the map Nate had tucked away in his duffel bag. Nate assured the men it must be somewhere between the Texas border and Mexico City, because that was where the map seemed to indicate most people in Mexico lived. But they could find no Gtz. between Texas and Mexico City. Slowly they scanned farther and farther down the map until they were at the bottom of Mexico where it borders Guatemala. There they found the province of Chiapas. And in the middle of Chiapas, they found the town of Tuxtla Gutierrez. On many maps, it turned out, the Gutierrez had been shortened to Gtz. Nate peered at the map, somehow hoping to get a clue as to what Tuxtla Gutierrez would be like. All he could see was a sea of unpronounceable place names, like Pijijiapan, Venustiano, and Huimanguillo.

In Laredo, Nate was going to collect a new propeller for the plane, but he hadn't thought much about carrying it across the border to Mexico. The propeller was seven feet long, hard to disguise, and not the kind of thing someone entering Mexico on a tourist visa normally carries. The Mexican border guards thought an airplane propeller was a strange tourist item, too, and they would not let him into Mexico with it.

Nate found a phone and called the CAMF headquarters office in Los Angeles to see what he should do about the problem. He was told to ship the propeller to Mexico City and, since time had been lost, catch a plane there himself. Nate was quite glad to be zipping through the air to Mexico City rather than rumbling along overland by train and bus.

In Mexico City, Nate was met by Betty Greene, who had flown up from Peru. She told him about the damage to the plane. Nate was stunned as he listened. What did she mean when she said he would find the two wings and the struts in baskets in the hangar at the Tuxtla airport? Surely they didn't make baskets big enough for airplane wings to fit in. As Nate was to find out soon enough when he peered into the hangar at Tuxtla, it all depends on how small the pieces of the wings are!

Propped up behind the baskets of wing pieces was what looked like a pile of junk. As he looked more closely, though, Nate discovered that the pile of junk was actually the wing struts and pieces of the landing gear that had been removed from the plane and brought eighty miles out of the jungle to Tuxtla. Standing in the hangar, surveying all the pieces, Nate knew he was going to be in Tuxtla Gutierrez for a very long time.

Nate walked around and tried to imagine how he would tackle the job. He thought about the model planes he'd made as a boy. Perhaps he could approach the job the same way as building a model. In fact, the Waco biplane wasn't a lot different from the models he had made. It was constructed mostly of wood and fabric; it was just a lot bigger than his model planes, and it had a real engine. He plotted out a plan to rebuild the plane. First he would make new wing parts from wood. Then he would concentrate on the struts and the wing root that held the wings to the fuselage of the airplane. Finally, he would fix the landing gear. By then, the propeller should have arrived, and he would take it and all the other parts to El Real in the jungle and assemble the wings there. The wings would be much too big to carry in one piece if he assembled them in Tuxtla.

The trouble was, Nate was a mechanic, not a woodworker. To get the job done, he would need to find a cabinetmaker who could also build airplane wing parts. But how could he find such a person when he couldn't even speak the language? He had been working hard on learning Spanish and could count to thirteen with confidence, but he was a long way from being able to tell someone what he wanted them to do. While his Spanish had a way to go, he could draw simple pictures, which he figured anyone could understand. So with notebook in hand, he drew pictures of a man who worked with chisels and saws and went off to find such a man who wanted a job making parts for an airplane. It was an overwhelming task, but amazingly, Nate came back to his one-room house with Santiago, who had immediately understood what Nate wanted done. Santiago was also a good cabinet-maker who learned well from pictures, and he didn't mind giving up building cabinets for a while to repair airplane wings.

The slow process of rebuilding the wings began. Nate and Santiago began working in the hangar, but the owner wouldn't let them use their tools inside the hangar. It was too hot and rainy to do the work outside, so there was only one thing to do. The two men moved their wing-building operation to Nate's one-room house. There wasn't much space to spare once the two men and the two wings were inside. The house itself was made of adobe brick with a tile roof. It had a front and a back door, but no windows. The doors themselves were constructed in two halves, much like barn doors. It didn't take Nate long to find out why they were like that. Without the doors open, the room had no sunlight. When the doors were wide open, there was plenty of sunlight, but pigs, chickens, and burros would then wander through the house to see what the two men were up to. An answer to the problem was soon discovered. With the top half of the door open and the bottom half closed, there was still plenty of sunlight to work by, but the visiting animal problem was solved.

There were other animal problems, though. Bats, rats, scorpions, and cockroaches all vied for living space in the rafters of the house. They were impossible to get rid of. At first Nate hunted them down, but as quickly as he did, more came flooding in to fill up the empty accommodation space in the rafters. He learned to be very thankful for his mosquito net, which he tucked tightly around his bed each night. The net formed a kind of boundary between his world and the world of rodents, bats, and bugs that took over the little house each night after dark.

Not only were the insects and animals a trial, but Nate also found the local food very strange. He thought of the many other uses there must be for tortillas, which tasted to him like cardboard. When he ate frijoles and the hot sauce that seemed to smother everything, his stomach revolted. In the end, his stomach would allow him to eat only tomatoes, boiled eggs, and bananas. Despite the food and the creatures in the rafters, Nate kept on working.

Each day, Nate took out the blueprints and worked on the wings, using the wood parts Santiago had crafted. He often worked late into the night. Finally, though, the heat, poor food, lack of sleep, and stress of the whole project combined to keep him in bed. He was very sick, but he didn't know what he was sick with, and there were no doctors around to tell him. His only information came from a basic medical handbook that Betty Greene had given him. Nate lay on his stomach and propped the book on his pillow. Somehow he had to figure out what was wrong with him. He started at 'A' and read all the symptoms for every illness until he got to 'J,' where he found the word *jaundice* and a list of symptoms. Weakness? Yes. He could hardly drag himself from his bed to the cactus bush outside that he used as a bathroom. Yellow coloring of the eyeballs? He reached for the mirror he kept on the shelf above his bed and pulled down his lower left eyelid. There was a definite yellow tinge in his eyes. As he read through the list, he discovered just how sick he was. He needed help, and he needed it fast. He pushed the medical handbook from his pillow, rolled onto his back, and began to pray.

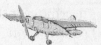

Chapter 6

The Remarkable Repair Job

The answer to Nate's prayer for help came in the form of Phil Baer, a missionary with Wycliffe Bible Translators. Phil was passing through Tuxtla on his way back to his mission station deep in the jungle, far beyond El Real where the Waco biplane had crashed. He was curious when someone in town told him about the American who was building wings in his house for a missionary airplane. Phil had to check it out, so he followed the directions to Nate's tiny adobe house. There he found a skinny man lying half conscious in bed, with airplane wing parts and a variety of tools spread around the room.

Immediately, he could see that Nate was in trouble. He radioed his mission station and told them he would be delayed in Tuxtla for a while. Then he set to work. First, he had to help Nate get well again. He concentrated on finding good food Nate could keep down. He went to the market each morning and bought meat and vegetables to make soup. Then he tackled the huge mound of dirty clothing and bedding that had piled up in Nate's house. There was no washing machine, so Phil had to wash everything by hand. To dry the laundry, he spread it on the cactus plant outside the house.

With good food and care, Nate's health quickly began to improve. Before long, Nate was up and about again. Phil insisted on staying to help Nate until he had finished making the parts for the wings. Phil lived in the jungle and knew how important it was for CAMF to be successful. The plane would save missionaries hundreds of hours of traveling time and would open up whole new areas to the gospel message.

The days rushed by. Phil took over all the household chores, from washing the laundry by hand to cooking on a camp stove. There wasn't much cleaning to do because the cactus bush outside the house was not only the clothesline but also the bathroom, and the shower consisted of three crates stacked outside the front door with a hose draped over the top of them. The crates were only shoulder high, and when he'd first arrived, Nate had been too embarrassed to shower during the day, waiting instead until nightfall. But as he quickly found out, even in southern Mexico it could get cold at night.

After a few weeks of shivering in the shower, he decided to start showering in the middle of the day with the sun beating steadily on his back and the occasional neighbor chatting with him as he soaped up.

Nate was grateful for Phil Baer's help. He realized that Phil had more important things to do than help a mechanic build airplane wing parts. But Phil never complained about the boring jobs or long hours he put in helping Nate, not to mention the time he was spending away from his wife and new baby. It was Nate's first experience with a real missionary in the field, and he was impressed with what he saw.

Time, though, was running out for Nate. He had only a couple of weeks left on his tourist visa and had to get the job finished. He had ordered the central beam that ran the length of the wing—the spar—and the wing root that connected the upper wing to the fuselage of the plane, but so far only the spar had arrived in Tuxtla. While he waited, Nate had a big problem to solve. As he studied the instructions that came with the spar, explaining in diagram form how it attached to the wing root, he noticed that the drawing of the wing root was different from the drawing on his blueprints. One of the drawings had to be wrong, but which one? Nate knew if he got to the jungle with the wrong wing root he would have to come all the way back to Tuxtla to make another one. That would waste days, and he didn't have days to spare.

Nate sat in front of his adobe house in the morning sun and thought about the problem. The only sensible thing to do, he decided, was to reconstruct the old wing root from the basket of pieces from the crash. He would then be able to compare it to the two different drawings to see which one was right. It took more than a day to sort out the splintered pieces that belonged to the upper wing and fit them back together into a spar and a wing root. Nate wondered as he worked which picture of the wing root would be the right one. The answer, he soon discovered, was neither. The reconstructed wing root was unlike either of the drawings; it was a completely different design!

Unfortunately, the broken pieces couldn't be fit back together accurately enough for Nate to use the old wing root as a pattern from which to make a new one. All he could do was take the materials to construct a new wing root into the jungle with him. There he could use the wing root from the right side of the plane as his pattern for the new one.

Finally, Nate had done all he could in Tuxtla. He needed to find the Waco biplane in the jungle and finish the repairs where it had crash-landed. But to get the eighty miles to the airstrip at El Real, he needed a plane that could transport him and all his parts and equipment. Since Phil could speak Spanish, he set off to see what he could find. Some locals told him about a charter plane that flew into town from time to time. Fortunately, the plane had just arrived a few days earlier.

Nate and Phil hunted all over Tuxtla for its owner. They found him in a tavern. He was a six-foot-two-inch, blond Dutchman named Hank. Unfortunately, Hank was too drunk to talk to, so Nate and Phil decided to come back the next day. But when they found Hank the next day, he was in a bad mood from being drunk the night before and didn't want to talk to anyone. It took several days of visiting Hank, and agreeing to pay him far too much money, to get him to fly Nate to El Real.

Dealing with a drunk, grumpy, greedy pilot opened Nate's eyes. *Is this what missionaries have to go through every time they need to get somewhere quickly?* Nate wondered. *How would I feel if it took two days to round up a pilot to fly my sick child to a hospital from some remote jungle location? An airplane could mean the difference between life and death.* Like never before, Nate understood the importance of airplanes in missionary work. He just hoped everything went well at El Real and he could get the Waco biplane flying again soon.

Early the next morning, Nate and Phil arrived at the airport complete with tools, blueprints, spars, the seven-foot propeller, and all the wooden wing parts Nate and Santiago had made. Nate had weighed every piece and had given Hank the weights. Hank didn't seem worried about how much the cargo weighed; he assured them there would be room for everything. Nate and Phil pushed and twisted and adjusted all the pieces until everything was stowed inside the plane. Nate thought it all looked too heavy for the Norseman airplane, but Hank was the pilot, and it was the pilot's job to know what was safe for his plane. *Besides,* Nate reassured himself, *Hank must know what he's doing or he wouldn't have survived as a jungle pilot.*

Nate held onto that thought as he climbed into the Norseman. He waved good-bye to Phil, who had been such a help and friend. By the time the Waco biplane was in the air again, Phil would be back home at his mission station with his family. Hank pushed the starter button, and the Norseman's engine belched into motion in a cloud of oily smoke. Nate cocked his head to listen. The engine sounded fine to his mechanic's ears.

Hank set the flaps for take-off and revved the engine, and the plane moved forward. He guided the plane to the end of the grass runway, turned it around, checked his instruments one last time, and pushed the throttle all the way forward. They rumbled down the runway. Nate noticed that with the load, the plane took a long time to gather speed. When one of its wheels hit a large mud puddle, the plane slowed. Nate waited for Hank to ease off the throttle and come around for another try at take-off, since there wasn't enough runway left to get airborne. But Hank didn't flinch. He looked straight ahead as the plane ploughed on down the runway, despite the fact it showed no signs of leaving the ground. Eventually, though, the wheels thumped heavily several times and then lifted off the ground. They were airborne, but the trees at the end of the runway were too close to clear. Nate could see Phil running toward the trees, and he wondered why. It wasn't until several years later when he met Phil again that he found out. Phil could see the trouble the Norseman was having getting airborne, and he was running toward the spot where he was sure it would crash. But somehow it didn't crash. An unexpected headwind helped the plane to barely clear the trees and gain altitude.

Nate's heart was pounding. They hadn't hit the trees. They were still airborne and heading east toward El Real. Nate looked across at Hank, who was still looking straight ahead. He began to wonder if he'd been wrong about Hank. Perhaps it wasn't good piloting skills that had kept him alive this long. And they still had to land! Nate began praying hard as lush green tropical vegetation passed beneath them.

The jungle was so thick that Nate didn't notice the El Real airstrip until they were right over it. Hank buzzed the strip with the Norseman as Nate peered down. He could make out the outline of the Waco biplane. Its nose and left side were covered with a blanket. Nate wondered what the damage looked like beneath the blanket.

Hank banked the plane around and came in for a steep landing. When the wheels hit the ground, Nate breathed a prayer of thanks and hoped he never had to be at Hank's mercy again.

Hank was eager to get back to Tuxtla, so he helped Nate unload the plane. As soon as the plane was empty, he was on his way, leaving Nate alone in the jungle. Nate didn't have time to think about the snakes or the jaguars that could be lurking in the trees around him; he had a job to do. He pulled the blanket off the fuselage. His heart sank when he saw the damage. The wing area was more torn up than he'd thought it would be.

Nate wondered if the engine would still run after sitting out for so long. He turned the key, which had been left in the plane, and hit the starter button; the engine sprang to life. That was one less thing Nate had to worry about fixing. That is, until it spluttered and died two minutes later. Nate frowned and wondered why it had stopped. He found the answer soon enough. Mud wasps had built little mud villages in the fuel tank and fuel lines. Nate would have to think of a way to get rid of them and then scrape out their homes. It took him a day to do it and get the engine running again.

More days were spent fitting the wings together and measuring the right wing root as a pattern for the left one, which he made on the spot. The wing pieces fit together as easily as his model airplanes had. Soon Nate was in the final stages of the repair work. He had brought cloth with him to patch the fuselage, but the hole was much bigger than he'd thought, and the cloth wouldn't be enough. So one of the last things he did was to rip up his sheets and use them to patch the last hole in the fuselage.

Nate was putting the finishing touches on the patch when he heard a plane overhead. It was Hank and the Norseman. The plane circled a couple of times before coming in for a landing. It stopped at the end of the airstrip just long enough for a tall, dark-haired man to climb out. As soon as the man was clear of the plane, Hank hit the throttle and was off again. The man strode over to Nate, shook his hand, and introduced himself as George Wiggins, the man who had been copilot of the Waco biplane when it crashed. Wiggins ran his hand over the repaired wing and whistled with admiration at the remarkable repair job Nate had done.

Later that day, George Wiggins and Nate loaded up Nate's tools and belongings, and then the Waco skipped down the runway with Wiggins at the controls. Nate had wanted to take the first flight alone, but the instructions from CAMF headquarters made it clear that George Wiggins was the official CAMF pilot, and he must be in the plane at all times. Nate decided he would have to say something about the situation to Jim Truxton and CAMF when he got back to the United States. It was an unacceptable risk sending up two men on a test flight.

Despite Nate's feelings about the unnecessary risk involved in the flight, the Waco lumbered into the air. The men flew around the tiny airstrip several times, reasoning that if anything went wrong, they had a better chance of landing again than if they were flying over dense jungle. Satisfied that the repairs were safe and the left wing wasn't going to fall off in flight, they pointed the nose of the Waco towards Tuxtla, leaving El Real behind. On the flight back, George Wiggins took his hands from the control wheel. The plane kept flying in a perfectly straight line, not veering to the right or the left. Nate heaved a sigh of relief; he had done a good job. There was no drag, and everything was in proper alignment.

The next morning, Nate was again relieved when he heard the biplane buzz over his hotel before it headed back to Mexico City and on to missionary service. The job was finished, and it was time for Nate to return to Los Angeles to report to CAMF.

When he got to Los Angeles, Nate found that CAMF had just changed its name to Missionary Aviation Fellowship (MAF). The report Nate gave to Jim Truxton and the MAF board helped fix in place many of the new mission's policies. Because Nate had done such a great repair job under difficult conditions, MAF decided that in the future, it would look for pilots who were also mechanics, or at least had knowledge of how to fix a plane.

Nate also pointed out MAF's need for lighter airplanes. If a lighter plane than the Waco had flown onto the El Real airstrip, it would have cleared the trees and not crashed. MAF had to stop taking the first or cheapest airplanes it was offered and instead choose planes that were useful and safe to fly in the jungle. Nate also explained that light planes are easier to fix when something goes wrong.

Finally, Nate talked about safety procedures. Everyone knew the risks of traveling by plane in the jungle, but why risk more lives than necessary? Nate described how he and George Wiggins had both flown in the Waco on its test flight. If something had gone wrong with the repairs and the plane had crashed, two lives would have been lost. The leaders of MAF agreed, and new safety rules were drawn up.

When Nate had finished his report, the MAF board asked him what his plans were for the future. He'd had a long time to think about this on the nights when the rats scurrying above his head had kept him awake. He knew what he wanted to do next, and he told the board, "I feel led to get additional schooling—so that I might be first a witness of His saving grace and then an airman." With that remark, it was settled. Nate would go to Wheaton College and then join MAF as a missionary pilot.

When Nate left the MAF office late in the day, there was one other thing he needed to do before leaving California. He needed to visit Marjorie Farris, the nurse he'd met while stationed in Merced. They had been writing to each other, and he had been wondering if a girl like Marj had ever dreamed of a little house in the jungle complete with rats, scorpions, and snakes. It was a long shot, he had to admit, but it couldn't hurt to ask!

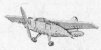

Chapter 7

Follow the Oil

Nate laid down his hammer and wiped his sweating brow. He poured himself a cup of water from a bottle perched on a log and looked around him. He never imagined Ecuador would be this beautiful. *No matter how long I live here*, he thought, *I will never get tired of the view.* To the south, about forty miles away, stood the snow-covered peak of Mt. Sangay, an active volcano. Every morning the mountain seemed different. Some mornings its top glowed red with lava, other mornings, smoke and ash billowed from it, blanketing the land below in grayness. To the east was jungle that stretched farther than the eye could see, all the way across the Amazon Basin to the Atlantic Ocean two thousand miles away.

Nate smiled to himself. The house he was building had a living room that faced Mt. Sangay. He could just see Marj and himself enjoying a morning cup of coffee as they admired the mountain's snow-capped peak.

Nate wondered how Marj was doing in Quito, the capital of Ecuador, high in the Andes Mountains more than a hundred miles to the north. He hoped she was getting plenty of rest; she deserved it. Ever since their wedding eight months earlier on Valentine's Day, February 14, 1948, they had been in a whirlwind of activity. First there had been the meetings with Missionary Aviation Fellowship to make sure they felt called by God to go out as MAF missionaries. Then there were all the meetings to raise money and explain the ministry of MAF. The whole idea of pilots being missionaries was new to many folk in the church. Nate liked to explain that the mission of MAF was not to do what commercial airlines could do more cheaply but to go where there were no other airlines and where missionaries needed them most. He would say, "Our responsibility is to harness aviation to the needs of the mission field."

Many churches and individuals had understood how useful an air service would be to missionaries and agreed to support Nate and Marj as they established MAF in Ecuador.

As soon as Nate had agreed to join MAF, Jim Truxton had set about finding the right location to

base the new ministry. He had studied a map of
Ecuador. The whole country is about the same size
as the state of Nevada. To the west, the country borders the Pacific Ocean. On the coastal lowlands
between the ocean and the Andes, bananas were
grown for export. Also on the lowlands and all the
way up to Quito, located high in the Andes
Mountains in the northcentral part of the country,
the roads were numerous and in fairly good condition. It was obvious there wasn't a particular need
for MAF there. But across the Andes in the eastern
part of the country, the roads were scarce and in terrible condition. This part of the country, called the
Oriente, forms the western edge of the Amazon rain
forest. Across the region, missionaries seeking to
share the gospel message with the many Indian
tribes that inhabited the area lived in stations dotted throughout the jungle. There was a great need
for more missionaries in the Oriente. The trouble
was, it was difficult traveling through the swampy
jungles to set up more mission stations. As Jim
Truxton looked at his map, he decided this was the
area where MAF needed to be working. The ministry would establish a base of operations in the
Ecuadorian Oriente.

Missionaries, however, were not the only West-
erners in the Oriente. There was another group of
people busy making roads and airstrips to support
their exploration of the area. This group of people
worked for Shell Oil Company and since 1938 had

been exploring the jungle looking for oil. Shell Oil had spent about forty million dollars developing the roads and airstrips necessary to carry men and supplies in and out of the Oriente. It had cost this much because the ground was covered with enormous trees such as balsa, ironwood, and mahogany. Once bulldozers cleared away the trees for a road or airstrip, the problem of the wet soil had to be overcome. Because the Oriente received more than three hundred inches of rain a year, the ground hardly ever dried out. And because it was so wet, the soil was unable to support the weight of a truck or a large aircraft landing. Tons of rock were blasted from the sides of nearby mountains and used to make foundations on the wet soil. On top of these foundations, the road or airstrip could be safely built. It was a long, expensive process, but Shell Oil was certain there were billions of gallons of oil beneath the jungle. All the work would be worth it if they could be the ones to pump the oil out of the ground.

Jim Truxton visited Shell Oil's largest airfield and the company's Ecuador headquarters. It was located several miles from the old village of Mera, and so was called Shell Mera. There Jim talked to the chief of operations and explained MAF's goals. He asked if Shell Oil would let a MAF plane use the airstrip. The chief of operations listened carefully and then explained that another plane to help out in an emergency would always be welcome at

Shell Mera, but he was worried about safety. If a MAF pilot crashed in the jungle, they would all have to take time out to look for him, and in many cases, planes that crashed in the jungle were never found.

Jim Truxton thought for a few moments, and then he made a deal with the chief of operations. MAF would rent an acre of land at the east end of the airfield for one dollar a year on the condition that the plane would have a radio on board and the pilot would stay in constant contact with an operator on the ground. That way, if the plane crashed, they would know where to look.

So the Missionary Aviation Fellowship followed Shell Oil Company into the Oriente, grateful for the hard work and money already spent to prepare the land for oil exploration that would now also be used to bring the gospel message to people who had never heard it.

Nate stripped off his shirt and went back to work, thankful that he was not building the new MAF house at Shell Mera alone. Charles Mellis Sr., a seventy-year-old builder from St. Louis, had come down to Ecuador to head up the building project. Jim Truxton was also there, as well as several missionaries whom Nate was going to be serving with his plane. Among them was Frank Drown, who would become one of Nate's lifelong friends.

Nate glanced across at the Stinson aircraft sitting just off the end of the runway. He may not have a house yet, but he did have an airplane. It had been the private plane of the owner of the Weyerhaeuser Company. When the owner heard about the work of Missionary Aviation Fellowship, he donated the plane for use in South America. Jim Truxton and Nate had flown it down from the United States. Now it sat on a runway in the jungle of South America, painted yellow, the color of MAF aircraft, and ready for whatever need came along.

In fact, Nate had already used the plane for the purpose it had been donated. Frank Drown, who had walked for seven days across jungle trails to help Nate build the house, mentioned that his family hadn't had any fresh food or medicine for five months. When he heard this, Nate took immediate action. As Frank dug foundation holes for the house, Nate flew out to Macuma Base, where Frank and his family were stationed, and dropped a supply of fresh food and a letter from Frank. As he banked around, Nate saw Frank's wife, Marie, waving her thanks for the food. He wished there was some way to ask her if everything was all right and to take a message back to Frank, but there wasn't. There was no radio at Macuma Base and no place nearby to land. As he flew back to Shell Mera, Nate marveled how in just thirty-seven minutes he had covered the same distance that had taken Frank seven days to walk.

The day after the flight to Macuma Station, another family needed Nate's help. The Coopers

were missionaries with the Christian and Missionary Alliance and needed transportation back to
their jungle home at Dos Rios. Mrs. Cooper much
preferred the idea of riding home in an airplane to
the way she had ridden out of the jungle. She had
come down with a bad case of malaria and needed
hospital treatment. The nearest hospital was at
Shell Mera, and having no other way to get there,
she had been carried all the way by a faithful
Indian guide! Now, three weeks later, she had
recovered enough to be out of the hospital, but it
would be months before she could face the walk
back to Dos Rios. Nate offered to fly her and her
family home, and in just over half an hour, they
were back among the Jivaro Indians. News spread
quickly among the missionaries of the Oriente that
Nate Saint and his yellow Stinson airplane were an
answer to prayer.

After Nate had been building the house at Shell
Mera for three weeks, he received some wonderful
news. Marj was coming to visit! She was six
months pregnant, and because things had not gone
well so far with the pregnancy, she had stayed
behind in Quito. She was staying at a guest house
run by HCJB, a radio ministry that broadcasted
Christian programs around the world. The guest
house was minutes away from the most modern
hospital in Ecuador. Despite the trouble Marj was
having with the pregnancy, her doctor had given
her permission to make the bumpy thirteen-hour

journey to visit Nate, as long as she lay down while she traveled.

Marj made the trip lying on a canvas cot in the back of a pickup truck. As she jostled along the winding road from Quito to Shell Mera, Nate prayed that she and the baby would be okay. They were. Marj climbed down from the truck a little wobbly on her legs but very grateful to have made it in one piece. Finally, she got to be with Nate in Ecuador. They had so much to talk about. During the evenings, they sat around the open fire, their backs to the army tents they slept in, and talked about their future. It was so exciting to be on the mission field, and Marj couldn't wait for the day when their baby would be born and she could move down to Shell Mera for good. But for now, they had to make the most of their week together.

Marj told Nate everything the doctor had said about how the pregnancy was progressing and all about her Spanish language lessons. Nate eagerly told her about his first local "ministry" opportunity. He had started a Sunday school for the children of Shell Mera. He told Marj how a week after they had begun building the house, two little girls from the Shell Oil base came and asked when Sunday school would be starting. It was too good an opportunity to miss, so Nate had immediately said to the girls, "It will be right here in this tent on Sunday morning." When Marj moved to Shell Mera for good after the baby was born, she and Nate would have an English-speaking Sunday school to run.

Nate also told Marj about the two flights he'd already made, and how he wished he could communicate with the missionaries on the ground. He then went on to tell her about their new "neighbors" in the jungle. Nate had first heard about them from David Cooper when he'd flown him and his wife and family back to Dos Rios. David had told Nate they were a tribe the local Quichua Indians called the "Aucas." In the Quichua language, Auca meant "savage," and the way David Cooper described them, the Aucas fit their name well.

White people had been in the jungles of Ecuador for three centuries, and in that time quite a few had met their death at the end of Auca spears. The first group into the jungle of the Oriente were Spanish explorers, then Catholic priests, and later on rubber hunters and gold prospectors. Finally had come oil companies searching for underground deposits of oil. Each group had stories to tell of ambush and terror that made the name Auca the most feared in all the Oriente. Members of other Indian tribes in the area knew the boundaries of Auca territory well: the Napo River to the north, the Villano River to the south, the Arajuno River to the west, and the Peruvian border to the east. It was nearly impossible to tempt anyone to cross over into Auca territory.

Nate told Marj all he'd heard from other missionaries about how the Aucas lived. They never wore clothes except for a woven string around their waist like a necklace. No one could be sure where they were at any time because they moved around a lot. They did not seem to have permanent houses or cultivate their land.

On the long evenings during Marj's stay at Shell Mera, Marj and Nate often prayed for the Aucas, who had never heard the gospel message and wouldn't unless something happened to change the way they "welcomed" outsiders. Somehow, Nate had a feeling his airplane would play a part in reaching them with the gospel; he just didn't yet know how it would all fit together.

The day before Marj was due to make the grueling trip back to Quito, she got to see firsthand the value of a pilot and airplane in the jungle. She was hoisting up a GI sheet to Nate, who was standing on the roof joists, when an Indian man came running out of the jungle. Out of breath, he handed a note to Marj. A little surprised, she opened it and read the scrawled writing: "Nancy Cooper sustained a bad gash."

Nate and Marj immediately went to work. Marj headed for the Shell clinic, while Nate climbed down from the roof and set about preparing the plane for flight. Half an hour later, he was in the air headed for the Dos Rios mission station with anti-tetanus serum and bandages aboard the plane.

Nate and the yellow MAF Stinson airplane were a blessing to so many people. But as Nate was about to find out, being a blessing could also be very dangerous. A pilot flying a plane over the

jungle is never more than a minute away from dis-
aster and death.

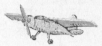

Chapter 8

A Perfect Take-Off...

The air was crisp and clear. It was the day before New Year's Eve, 1948, and Nate was whistling to himself as he loaded up the Stinson aircraft. As he positioned suitcases and boxes, he couldn't help thinking about Marj. He had just come from the guest house where she was staying in Quito, and the good news was that everything with the pregnancy was fine and the baby was due any day now, maybe even on New Year's Day. *That would be an easy birthday to remember,* Nate thought. Once the Stinson was loaded, Mrs. Tidmarsh and her twelve-year-old son, Bob, were ready to board the plane. Nate helped Mrs. Tidmarsh into the backseat of the plane. Bob, holding a bag of candies, climbed into the front seat. Nate smiled to himself as he saw the look of excitement in Bob's eyes. It reminded him of how he'd been when he took his first flight with Sam.

Nate buckled his seat belt across his lap and made sure his two passengers did the same. He cranked the Stinson's engine to life, looked over his gauges, and then checked to make sure his flaps and ailerons were working properly. He set the flaps for take-off. There was no one at the airfield to wave good-bye to them, so Nate revved the engine and taxied to the end of the runway. As he positioned the plane for take-off, he checked the wind sock. It was almost still except for a slight crosswind from the east. Nate gunned the engine, and the Stinson headed down the runway for a perfect take-off.

Although located 9,300 feet above sea level, Quito is in a big valley surrounded by high snow-covered peaks. Nate looked at the mountains he would have to gain altitude to cross. As the Stinson vibrated with the engine at full throttle, he looked at the altimeter to check his rate of ascent out of Quito. He was two hundred feet off the ground and beyond the boundary of the Quito airfield. Below were cultivated fields. Nate glanced across at Bob, whose eyes were as big as saucers as he took everything in.

Suddenly, from nowhere, a violent downdraft slammed into the Stinson. The bag of candies Bob was holding flew out of his hand, and the suitcases in the luggage compartment at the back were hurled against the roof of the plane. Nate knew they were in trouble. He didn't have enough altitude to contend with a downdraft this strong. He jerked the control wheel to keep the wings level as he tried to maneuver out of the unusually strong air current. But the airplane was dropping too fast. It was plummeting, and there was nothing he could do to stop it. The last thing Nate remembered was a plowed field rushing up to meet the Stinson.

Nate opened his eyes and squinted at the bright light. He was in a large room with tiled walls, and people were moving around him. He heard voices. "Give him ten more milligrams of morphine," someone said. The words seemed to float by him. He felt a prick in his arm, and then everything went blank.

Later—Nate had no idea how much later—he opened his eyes again. This time he was in a smaller room, and Marj was standing over him. As he moved, she patted him on the hand. "Try not to move," she said. But he couldn't have moved even if he had wanted to. His body, from neck to hips, was encased in a giant plaster cast. His left foot was also in a cast. Marj told him he had a compression fracture of his fourth lumbar vertebra and a severely pulled ligament in his left ankle. His back was going to take a long time to heal. Nate asked about his passengers, and Marj told him Mrs. Tidmarsh had broken the small bones in both lower legs, and Bob had escaped with only bumps and bruises. Both of them would make a full recovery.

Marj, who had thought Nate would be visiting *her* in the hospital any day soon, was now in charge of a badly injured husband. At that moment, Nate was glad she'd become a nurse instead of the mathematics teacher she'd set out to be. After talking at length with the doctors in Quito, Marj told Nate that they weren't sure how best to treat his injuries and that he ought to go back to the United States to be treated by a North American doctor with more experience in this type of injury.

Nate's heart sank; they didn't have the money for him to fly home. But Marj was one step ahead of him. Before he sank into depression over the situation, she reminded him he was an army veteran and, as such, he could get treatment at any army hospital free of charge. There was a large military hospital at the United States base in Panama, and Marj had already made arrangements for Nate to be flown there. The U.S. military had a cargo plane stationed in Quito that would ferry Nate to the hospital in Panama for treatment. Because Marj's pregnancy was too far advanced for her to travel, she would stay in Quito and have the baby.

With a cast covering half his body, Nate looked like a mummy as he was carried on a stretcher to the military transport plane. As he crossed the tarmac to the plane, he caught a glimpse of the yellow Stinson, which lay in a crumpled heap in front of a hangar where it had been dragged. The fuselage was broken in half, and the engine and landing gear had been ripped right off the plane. As he looked at the wreckage, Nate knew it was a blessing that he was alive.

On the flight to Panama, Nate had to stay lying on his back on the stretcher, since his cast didn't bend at the waist. He passed the time counting the number of rivets in the bulkhead. It was frustrating for him to be only a few feet from the cockpit and not be able to go up front and visit with the flight crew.

At the hospital in Panama, a battery of tests were run on Nate. After reviewing the results, the doctors decided his cast was immobilizing the wrong part of his back. The old cast would need to be cut off and a new one put on. That was the bad news. The good news arrived on January 10, 1949, the day after he arrived in Panama. It came in the form of a telegram from Quito, and it read, "Kathy Joan Saint born January 9th. All is well. Love Marj." Nate let out a whoop of joy. Everything was fine; he was now a dad! He wrote straight back to Marj and said, "Honey, don't be afraid to give that little gal lots of loving. She'll need the practice for when her daddy gets home....May the Lord guide our steps until we are making footprints side by side again."

As he lay in his hospital bed, Nate played the accident over and over again in his mind. There were so many questions that needed answers: How had it happened? What could be done to stop it happening again? How had the 9,300-foot elevation affected things? Obviously, the mountains around the airfield caused the wind to move in unusual patterns, and that was almost certainly the cause of the sudden downdraft. Still, if he'd had a bit more airspeed, the whole accident might never have happened. Letters between Nate and MAF headquarters in Los Angeles hashed over every detail of the short flight. Finally, everyone concluded that the sudden downdraft had caused the accident. But they also noted that in mountains at that elevation, downdrafts should be anticipated.

Nate also wondered whether there could have been some way to prevent his back from being broken. The lap belt had kept his hips in place, but the impact had flung the top half of his body forward, fracturing his back. What was needed were shoulder harnesses as well as lap belts. A shoulder harness would have held him in his seat and stopped him from being jerked around and injured more. Nate wrote to Jim Truxton and told him his thoughts on fitting shoulder' harnesses to MAF planes. Jim thought it was a good idea and ordered all MAF aircraft to be fitted with them immediately.

Nate spent a month at the hospital in Panama before doctors decided he was well enough to return to Ecuador. His back was healing nicely, but he had strict instructions from his doctors. He was to wear his cast for another five months and then have it cut off. After that time, he would have to wear a back brace, which the doctors made especially for him, until his back muscles were strong again. That would probably take another five months.

The military transport plane flew Nate back to Quito. This time, though, Nate got to stand up for the whole trip because of his new cast. It was tiresome standing for the whole flight. But despite his weary legs by the end of the journey, he couldn't wait to see Marj and new baby Kathy, who were waiting at the airport to meet him. His face beamed as he took his first look at the little blonde bundle Marj was carrying.

The newly enlarged Saint family spent several days in Quito. While there, HCJB, the ministry whose guest house Marj had been staying in, asked Nate to talk on the radio. The name HCJB was short for "Heralding Christ Jesus' Blessings," and the ministry's goal was to send Christian programming around the world by radio. Quito's high elevation and proximity to the equator meant there was little atmospheric interference of radio signals from the earth's magnetic field. Strange as it seemed, Quito, high in the Andes Mountains, was a perfect place from which to share the gospel message with the world.

During his many days in the hospital, Nate had been thinking about the idea of "expendability," and that was the subject of his radio talk. Expendability comes from the word *expend*, which means to use up. Nate used the term to mean that Christians need to offer themselves to be used up by God however He wishes to use them. During his talk, Nate said that "missionaries constantly face expendability. And people who do not know the Lord ask why in the world we waste our lives as missionaries. They forget that they too are expending their lives. They forget that when their lives are spent and the bubble has burst they will have nothing of eternal significance to show for the years they have wasted.

"Some might say, 'Isn't it too great a price to pay?' When missionaries consider themselves—their lives before God—they consider themselves expendable. And in our personal lives as Christians isn't the same thing true? Isn't the price small in the light of God's infinite love? Those who know the joy of leading a stranger to Christ and those who have gone to tribes who have never heard the gospel gladly count themselves expendable...."

Nate knew what he was talking about when he talked of expendability. He had nearly been killed in a plane crash. Yet it didn't deter him. He was ready to get back in an airplane and serve other missionaries.

Nate, Marj, and Kathy took the bus back to Shell Mera. Once again, Nate couldn't sit down for the trip. He spent the entire thirteen hours standing on the back bumper of the bus, clinging to a handrail! *If the doctors could see me now,* he thought, *they would never have released me.* Still, Nate quickly forgot about the discomfort of the journey as the bus rolled down the dusty road and the new house at Shell Mera came into view.

After thirteen hours on the bus, Nate and Marj were both a little wobbly. They staggered into the yard of their brown stained house, whose timber had been cut from trees that once grew where the house now stood. The aluminum roof glistened in the sun.

As they settled into their new home, Nate and Marj grew to love it. Marj enjoyed the sense of being almost outdoors, because the house had large open windows in every room covered only with screens. The house was also almost bug-free, because the foundations were concrete pillars, each with a moat around it filled with oil, barring entrance by termites and other insects. Of course, there were a few things the house didn't have, like electricity and running water. To take a bath, the Saints had to wait for rain. They never had to wait for long, though, because Shell Mera had more than thirty-two feet of rain a year. When it rained, they would gather up soap and a towel and head over to where the rainwater flowed off the edge of the runway. The water flowing into a ditch there made a good shower.

Nate was not the type to sit around, or stand around, as his cast forced him to do. With his cast still on, he managed to find plenty of jobs to keep himself busy. He dug post holes for a fence around the yard and laid gravel to make a taxiway from the airstrip to the hangar that had been built next to the house. Unfortunately, the hangar was empty, because there was still no replacement plane stationed at Shell Mera. Missionaries had to revert to hiking through the jungle for days to get where they wanted to go. When Nate heard about one such trip that nearly claimed the life of a missionary, he became concerned. Three missionaries had been trekking out from the isolated Macuma station. While crossing a turbulent river on a raft, they lost some of their equipment. Then one of the missionaries became violently ill from fatigue. Because their food rations were dwindling, he struggled on with the others. Their ordeal had lasted for six days. And when they finally reached Shell Mera, the one missionary's feet and legs were so swollen he could barely walk.

A replacement airplane was needed at Shell Mera, and it was needed fast. But before Nate could write to MAF to stress the urgency of the need, he received word from Jim Truxton in Los Angeles that a replacement plane was on its way to Shell Mera. Several days later, Hobey Lowrance, a MAF pilot sent to replace Nate until he was able to fly again, piloted the yellow, four-seater Piper Pacer across the Andes to Shell Mera, where he pulled it to a halt in front of the new hangar. Nate was waiting outside.

Hobey settled into the house with Nate and Marj. Soon he was busy servicing the missionary bases across the Oriente with the new plane. The missionaries were deeply grateful to again have air service to assist their work in the jungle.

Finally, five months passed, and it was time for Nate to take off the uncomfortable and, by now, very dirty cast. Marj walked with him to the Shell medical clinic. She carried with her the back brace that had been specially made for Nate in Panama. Nate would have to wear the brace right away because his back would be too weak and floppy for him to stand up without it. At least that's what the doctors thought.

After the cast was taken off, Nate walked home with his brace on. It felt just as uncomfortable as the cast had, but with one big difference: Nate could take the brace off if he wanted to. And that's exactly what he did. When he got home, he hung it up in the corner of his closet and never wore it again. His back wasn't weak and floppy at all. The digging and gravel laying he'd been doing had made it as good as new.

Now, with the accident finally behind him, Nate was eager to get back to flying. He had some new ideas he wanted to try out.

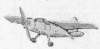

Chapter 9

Tin Can Lifesaver

Hobey Lowrance took Nate up for a checkout flight to certify that he was fit and ready to resume his flying duties. After he'd certified Nate to fly again, Hobey returned to the United States.

Finally, after surviving a difficult pregnancy and a broken back, Marj and Nate were on their own, and it felt good. One evening, not long after Hobey Lowrance had left, Marj fixed some lemonade and grabbed a handful of the peanut butter cookies she'd baked the night before, and she and Nate sat in the living room on the orange crates they used as chairs. Together they drank and talked and munched away. They chatted about the future and their life together at Shell Merita, the name they had given to the new house. Nate talked about how excited he was to be back flying. As he talked, the conversation slowly turned toward one of the problems that had bothered him before the crash in Quito.

"I've been thinking about the problem of communicating with missionaries on the ground," he began. "Those times when a missionary needs help and there is no airstrip for me to land or I'm running out of daylight and don't have the time to land and take off."

"What about your 'bombing' system?" Marj asked. She was referring to the device Nate had developed where items could be put into small cylinders on the wings of the plane, and when he pulled a rope in the cockpit, a hatch would open and the items would parachute to the ground.

"That's great for making medicine and mail drops, but what if the person on the ground needs to talk to me? I had a long time to think about this in the hospital, and I've got an answer. Get your sewing box and I'll show you."

Marj was used to Nate asking for strange things, so she brought him the sewing box. He placed it on the chest that served as a coffee table and opened it. He pulled out a reel of red thread and unwound about four feet of it. He tied the end of the thread to a pencil.

"Actually, I first thought about this during a church history class back at Wheaton College," he said with a grin. "Watch this." Nate stood up holding on to the reel, with the pencil swinging freely at the end of the thread. "What do you see?" he asked.

Marj looked puzzled. "A pencil swinging in a big circle," she replied.

Nate nodded. "And what about the reel of thread, what's it doing?"

Marj stared at the reel. "It's doing nothing," she said. "You're just holding it still in the middle, and the pencil is swinging around it in circles at the end of the thread."

"Exactly," said Nate with a smile. "Now think of it backwards."

Suddenly Marj could see what he was driving at. If it was turned upside down and the pencil was rotated in a circle around the outside of the reel, the reel would stand still in the center.

"Now imagine the reel is a supply bucket with a telephone in it, and the thread is a telephone wire."

"And if you fly in circles and drop the bucket down on the wire, then you think the bucket will eventually stay still in the middle of the circle?" Marj questioned.

"You got it," replied Nate, as he pulled a notebook from his pocket. "Now look at this."

Marj leaned over as Nate opened the notebook. Inside were a series of diagrams showing different weights, lengths of rope, and radiuses of circles.

"This will take a little working out, but I think I can design a system for dropping a telephone into the middle of the circle so I can use it to talk to missionaries on the ground," Nate said confidently.

The concept was so simple—it was just like the calm in the eye of a hurricane. Nate was amazed no one had thought of it before. He and Marj discussed how to test the idea. He would have to be sure the procedure was safe for both him and the person on the ground. After some practice to perfect the technique, Nate's "bucket drop" system proved to be a great success, and it wasn't long before it was used to save lives.

Frank Mathis, a missionary doing some Bible translation work in the area, received an urgent message from the Indians at nearby Arapicos. The whole village had been infected with a disease by some soldiers traveling through the area. One young warrior had already died, and unless Frank could help them, many others seemed doomed to die also. Frank Mathis immediately set off down the jungle trail to Arapicos while a fellow missionary with the Gospel Missionary Union, Bob Hart, contacted Nate to see if he had any ideas on how to help the situation.

It wasn't long before Nate and Bob Hart were winging their way over the jungle toward Arapicos. As they flew, Nate pointed out the canvas bucket and the fifteen hundred feet of telephone wire that lay on the back seat of the plane. He told Bob about his bucket system. A telephone was wrapped in a blanket in the canvas bucket. Nate explained that Bob would have to drop the bucket from the side of the plane and slowly let the wire out while Nate flew in circles. Bob wasn't sure he knew exactly what Nate meant, but there was no time for questions, because within a couple of minutes they were circling Arapicos.

At the sound of the plane, Frank Mathis came running out of one of the huts in the village. He stood in a clearing and waved frantically at the plane. Nate smiled; he knew what Frank was thinking. There was no airstrip and therefore no way for Frank to communicate with the plane.

Nate circled the Pacer over the clearing. He could almost see the puzzled look on Frank's face. Then he gave the signal to Bob to drop the bucket with the telephone in it from the side of the plane. The bucket trailed behind the plane, arcing down on the long telephone wire. When all the wire had been let out, Nate banked the Pacer more steeply and reduced the size of the circle he was flying in. As he did so, the bucket began to arc inwards until it hovered a few feet away from Frank.

Frank ran over to the bucket and grabbed it. He pulled the blanket out and found the telephone. He let out a yell in amazement. He lifted the phone to his ear and heard a crackling noise. Then loud and clear through the crackle he heard the words, "Hello, Frank, this is Bob Hart. What's the situation down there?"

"Pretty bad," announced Frank, the amazement of talking to the plane above him by phone sounding in his voice. "Most of the village is sick."

Nate had Bob find out from Frank what the symptoms of the sickness were. As Frank told him the symptoms, Bob hurriedly wrote them down. Then he handed the list to Nate, who tuned the plane's shortwave radio in to the hospital at Shell Mera, where a doctor was standing by, and relayed the list of symptoms over the radio. The doctor asked a few more questions, which were relayed by Bob down to Frank Mathis, and soon the doctor had all the information he needed to make a diagnosis. Bob pulled the bucket and telephone back onboard the Pacer, and the plane headed back for Shell Mera. By the time they landed, Marj was waiting with medicine to treat the illness. Nate refueled the airplane and flew back to deliver the lifesaving medicine.

That night as he drank his coffee with Marj, Nate explained the wonderful feeling of having saved lives without ever landing his plane. The bucket drop system had proved its usefulness.

News of Nate's ingenious maneuver with the bucket and wire spread around the world. He even received a surprise in the mail, a letter of commendation and 250 dollars from John Gaty, the general manager of the Beech Aircraft Company. Gaty was impressed with Nate's spiral-line technique, as it came to be known.

After the success of the bucket drop idea, Nate turned his attention to another problem. This time it was a safety issue. Flying over dense jungle, like that of the Oriente, was very dangerous, especially if something went wrong with the plane. On May 9, five months after the accident that nearly took his own life, Nate heard about a pilot and copilot from the Shell Oil Company who were killed while test-piloting a new Grumman airplane. Soon after that, an Ecuadoran transport plane crashed in the dense jungle. The crash site was only thirty-five miles from Shell Mera. All eleven passengers and crew were killed in the crash. Then in July, another Shell Oil Company plane flying passengers to the nearby town of Ambato crashed. Again, everyone on board was killed, thirty-eight passengers and crew in all.

Within six months of Nate's accident at Quito, fifty-one people lost their lives in airplane crashes within a hundred miles of Shell Mera. Each of the pilots in those planes had been more experienced than Nate. The crashes had given Nate a lot of reasons to think about safety when flying over the jungle.

Bob Hart, from the Gospel Missionary Union, was also a pilot, and he told Nate the story of what had happened to him about six months before Nate arrived at Shell Mera. Bob and George Poole, another missionary, had been flying over the jungle near Arajuno. They were cruising along about fifteen hundred feet above the jungle when the engine failed. They began to lose altitude, but there was nowhere to land. As far as the eye could see there was nothing except thick, green vegetation. Bob brought the plane down as best he could. While trying to avoid a huge balsa tree, the right wing clipped a palm tree, flipping the plane over as it crashed to the darkness of the jungle floor. The canopy of trees above them closed over the wreckage so that searchers couldn't see it from the air.

Bob had broken his ankle and shattered his knee and was unable to walk. George Poole was badly cut and bruised, but nothing was broken. They decided George would walk for help. For nine days, George wandered through the jungle, all the while wondering whether Bob was still alive. Finally, George made it to Shell Mera, but he was unable to locate exactly where the plane had crashed. It took another two days before Bob Hart, more dead than alive, was finally found. Bob lived to tell a story every jungle pilot knew could happen to him if his engine ever quit while flying over the jungle. Bob's story sent a chill up Nate's newly healed spine.

Apart from human error, where a pilot makes a major mistake or miscalculation while flying, the biggest concern to pilots was their airplane's engine quitting in midair. If a car's engine quits, the driver can coast to a halt at the side of the road, normally with no harm to anyone. But when a plane engine quits in midair, it's a different story. An airplane's propeller corkscrews through the air, pulling the plane along with it. As the plane is pulled forward, the movement of air over and under the wings creates lift, which keeps the plane aloft. When the engine stops, the propeller stops, the plane's forward motion quickly slows, and as it does, the lift under the wings is reduced and the plane begins to lose altitude. If a pilot is flying over an open field or a road when this happens, he might be able to glide the plane in for an emergency landing. But if he is flying over jungle, he can do nothing to avoid hitting the trees.

Nate thought hard about the things that were likely to make an engine quit in midair. It was hardly ever the engine itself that was the problem, since it was checked over before every flight. Ninety-nine percent of the time when an engine quit in flight it was because the fuel was contaminated or had stopped flowing to the engine. So Nate made a list of the ways that fuel was most likely to be stopped from reaching the engine. Number one on his list was mud wasps plugging up a fuel line, which is what had happened on the airstrip at El Real in Mexico. Number two was water in the fuel. Of course, this didn't actually stop fuel from reaching the engine; the fuel just didn't ignite when it got there. Number three was cracks in the fuel tank. Number four was dirt under the float valve seat. And number five was running out of fuel either because of a faulty gauge or because of human error.

Nate knew number five on his list was more common that any pilot liked to admit. Sometimes a pilot would change plans in the middle of a flight, or in an emergency a pilot would be tempted to take a risk and hope that there was enough fuel in the gas tank to make it the extra distance.

Nate felt there had to be some way to lessen the chance of an airplane engine's quitting over the jungle. But what was it? There were so many different ways the fuel supply could be cut off. He tried to come up with the answer, but nothing seemed to suggest itself as a solution. Then one day, as he worked away in the MAF hangar at Shell Mera, a truck went lumbering along the road on its way to Ambato. Lots of trucks passed Shell Mera on their way to Ambato, but something about this one caught Nate's attention. A boy was sitting on the roof of the truck cab with a five-gallon can of gas and a siphon tube. On the truck's fender beside the engine was another boy. He held the other end of the siphon tube. He tweaked the end of the tube with his fingers to control the flow of gas as he aimed it into the truck's air cleaner.

Nate laughed out loud when he realized what the boys were doing. With their tank of gas and siphon tube they were feeding fuel into the truck's carburetor in a tiny stream, completely bypassing the truck's own fuel storage system. It was a simple and ingenious trick, and it gave Nate inspiration. Why not use the same idea to bypass the fuel storage system of an airplane in an emergency?

Nate ran to the house and grabbed two of Marj's cooking oil cans. Back in the hangar, he beat them into the shape of a three-gallon tank and soldered them together. Then he cut a piece of balsa wood and shaped it into a cowling to go over the tank to make it aerodynamic. He strapped the tank and the cowling onto the left wing strut, and then he took a length of copper tubing and used it to connect the tank made from cooking oil cans to the manifold intake of the plane's engine. He put a valve on the end of the tubing and made a control rod from the valve to the instrument panel inside the plane. With the rod he could control the flow of fuel from the can to the engine.

It was dark by the time Nate finished his project, too dark to take the plane up for a test flight. So he put his tools away and headed to the house for dinner. All evening he thought of reasons why his new invention wouldn't work. After all, if the solution really was that easy, why hadn't someone thought of it before? And what if not enough fuel flowed through the copper tube and starved the engine, or too much flowed and flooded it?

By the next morning, Nate had almost reasoned himself out of taking the airplane up for a test flight—almost, but not quite. He tested the extra fuel tank in the hangar first. He started the engine and then gunned it before shutting it off and pulling the control rod he'd made the night before. When he shut it off, the engine didn't miss a beat as it changed from its own fuel supply to the one in the tin can strapped to its wing. The whole thing worked like a charm.

Still it was one thing for it to work while the plane was sitting still and level on the ground. Now Nate needed to know whether it would work in flight. He took off in the plane and circled Shell Mera about two thousand feet above the airstrip. Then Nate did the one thing that a pilot tries to avoid at all costs; he shut off the regular flow of fuel to the engine. Within a few seconds, the engine began to sputter. Nate reached down and pulled the control rod for his emergency device on the instrument panel, and the engine shuddered back to life. Twenty minutes later, the engine was still humming along on its emergency fuel supply. Nate tested the system every way he could think of. He banked sharply one way and then the other. He climbed rapidly and then put the plane into a dive. In every instance, the cooking oil can fuel tank worked perfectly, and the engine never once faltered.

Nate could hardly wait to land the plane and share his success with Marj. With just four pounds of added weight and less than a dollar's worth of parts, he had solved a problem that could save many lives in the jungle, maybe even his own.

He wrote to MAF headquarters in California about his invention. Jim Truxton agreed that it was a great safety improvement, and like Nate's suggestion about fitting shoulder harnesses, he ordered all MAF planes to be fitted with Nate's "tin can lifesaver." Nate also applied for a patent for his invention and approval for it from the Civil Aeronautics Authority. He received both.

Nate's mind was running in other directions, too. In 1949, some of the students in his Sunday school class told him they would be leaving Shell Mera. After eleven years at Shell Mera, Shell Oil Company had decided to stop any further exploration in the Oriente. There was certainly oil beneath the jungle, but the company had decided there wasn't enough oil for it to be a profitable operation.

Since Shell Merita and the MAF property were leased from Shell Oil Company, Nate and Marj wondered what would happen to them. In fact, they wondered what would happen to all the buildings at Shell Mera. If someone didn't use them, they would quickly be overrun by the jungle again. Nate and Marj discussed the situation and came up with a big plan. Why not have MAF buy the property that the house and hangar sat on, as well as the airstrip and a little extra land on each side. Then it could get one of the other missionary groups working in the area to buy the property with the other buildings on it. Nate discussed the idea with his friend Frank Drown, who was a missionary with the Gospel Missionary Union. Shell Mera, it turned out, was just the facility his mission needed for a planned Bible college to train local Indian Christians.

And so, the headquarters for Shell Oil Company's exploration of the Oriente became the permanent home of MAF and the Berean Bible Institute. The facility, which had cost Shell Oil Company more than sixty thousand dollars to establish, was sold to both groups for a tenth of its value. Nate and Marj couldn't have been happier. Things were going better than they could have possibly hoped.

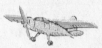

Chapter 10

Raising the Roof

Nate and his older sister Rachel had a lot to catch up on when she came to visit in mid-1951. Of course, the first thing Rachel wanted to do was see her new nephew, Steve, born to Marj and Nate in January 1951. Steve was a happy, bouncy boy, and he took an instant shine to his Aunt Rachel. As Rachel and Nate sat together in the evenings and sipped coffee or lemonade and watched Mt. Sangay's crater glowing in the distance, Nate told her all about his emergency fuel tank device and his bucket drop technique. Rachel laughed as she listened. Nate hadn't changed much from the little blond boy back in Huntingdon, Pennsylvania, full of dreams and schemes.

Rachel, in turn, told Nate all about her decision to become a Bible translator and about the two years she had worked among the Shapras Indian tribe in Peru. In 1948, at thirty-five years of age, Rachel had left the rescue mission in New Jersey where she had been working successfully with recovering alcoholics to become a missionary in the Amazon region. Her friends thought she was crazy, but deep inside, Rachel felt a call and a promise from God that centered around one verse: Romans 15:21. The verse said, "Those who have never been told of Him shall see and those who never heard shall understand." Rachel felt that God was calling her to make contact with a tribe which had never before heard the gospel message, and when she did make contact, she believed they would understand the message and respond to it.

After attending Wycliffe Bible Translator's jungle training camp in El Real, Mexico, near where Nate had repaired the crashed Waco biplane, Rachel had moved on to Peru. There she worked with two other Wycliffe missionaries translating the New Testament into the language of the Shapras Indians. It was challenging work, and Rachel loved it. But rewarding as the work was, somehow she felt it wasn't God's final destination for her. She felt there was another tribe God would lead her to, and there, amid that tribe, she would truly fulfill the promise from the verse in Romans.

Nate listened to all she had to say. Then several days later, when he took Rachel up flying with him, he flew out across the jungle before banking steeply to the left. As the plane turned, he motioned with his head in the direction of a ridge about ten miles away off the right side of the plane. "There's your tribe, Sis, just beyond that ridge," he said. He told her the little he knew about the Auca Indians. But Rachel was hardly listening; somehow she knew beyond a doubt that they were the people God was calling her to. She didn't know how it would happen, because Wycliffe Bible Translators didn't even work in Ecuador, but she knew God would arrange it. When Rachel returned to Peru and the Shapras Indians, she went back with a new excitement for all God had planned for her in the future.

By the time 1952 rolled around, Nate and Marj had been stationed at Shell Mera for three years, and it was time for them to take an extended break. MAF sent Bob and Keitha Wittig to take their place while they were away. After the Wittigs had settled in and Nate had oriented Robert to jungle flying and the locations of the various mission stations scattered across the Oriente, Nate and Marj gathered up three-year-old Kathy and one-year-old Steve and headed for the United States, where the kids would meet their grandparents for the first time.

Back in the United States, the Saints moved into a cottage on a missionary housing compound in Glendale, California. Grandma and Grandpa Farris, Marj's parents, moved into a house nearby. They, of course, were excited to be near their grandchildren. Having Marj's parents close by worked out well for

Nate and Marj, who were able to speak in churches or meet with MAF officials and know their children were well taken care of by their grandparents. It was also a great arrangement for the children, who were treated to many ice cream treats by their grandparents.

Their time in the United States rolled by quickly. Nate and Marj had many invitations to speak at churches across the country. Many people had heard stories of the "savage" tribes of the Amazon region, and they wanted to hear more about the region firsthand from frontier missionaries working there. Whenever the Saints spoke at a church, they made it a point to speak in the Sunday school as well. Nate and Marj both knew how important it was for young people to understand that God had a plan for their lives.

When Nate and Marj were not speaking at churches, Nate worked on new safety features for jungle planes. He was able to do this thanks to Granddad Proctor. His grandfather had died before Nate was born, but the money from his will wasn't distributed until 1952, when all his grandchildren came of age. Nate and Marj decided to do three things with the money they received. First, they put a little of it away as emergency money in case something happened to Nate and Marj had to raise the children alone. Second, they used much of it to buy the land around Shell Merita which they gave to MAF. Lastly, they kept some money aside so Nate could experiment with new safety features.

While Nate was busy with his experiments, Marj was out buying enough clothes to last them all until they came back to the United States on furlough again in another five years. It wasn't easy deciding what Kathy or Steve would like to wear, or even what size they would be in five years, but Marj guessed as best she could.

Nate kept in regular contact with the Wittigs at Shell Mera. The Wittigs were doing a fine job, but they were amazed at how much work Nate and Marj had to do. They understood why after three years the two of them had needed to take a break. They wrote to Jim Truxton and told him the work of MAF in Shell Mera was too much for one couple to do all by themselves. As a result, by the time Nate and Marj were ready to return to Ecuador in the spring of 1953, MAF had decided to send another couple to Shell Mera to work with the Saints. This also meant that another airplane was needed. Nate helped MAF choose a Piper Family Cruiser for the job. The Piper Cruiser had longer wings than the Pacer, which meant it could land on shorter airstrips. Nate thought it would be perfect for jungle flying.

Nate was very pleased with the way the Piper Cruiser performed as he flew his family across the United States from California to Huntingdon, Pennsylvania. He landed at the same airstrip where Sam had taken him up for his first flight twenty-three years before. Sam and most of the family were waiting for them at the old house. It was a proud moment for Nate to introduce his two children to all their aunts, uncles, and cousins. Of course, their time together went by too fast, and before long, Nate and a copilot from MAF were headed south over Mexico toward Ecuador in the Piper Cruiser. Marj and the children followed later by commercial airliner.

Seven days later, Nate flew over the patch of cleared Ecuadoran jungle he called home. He was glad to get back. As he circled the landing strip, he could see Bob and Keitha Wittig waving enthusiastically to him. It wasn't long before he was sitting in his own living room sipping lemonade and listening to Bob tell the story of his "unfortunate" adventure.

Just several days before, Bob had been delivering a load of building materials to the Dos Rios missionary base. He was hurtling down the Shell Mera airstrip at full throttle for take-off when a huge dog began racing across the airstrip toward the plane. Bob could see it getting closer and closer, so he pulled on the control wheel and tried to get the plane off the ground. He didn't have quite enough speed, so the plane responded slowly. Bob heard a heart-sickening thud, and he knew the dog had hit the plane. He managed to get the plane into the air and then began to scramble for what to do next.

Nate leaned forward, waiting to hear what happened next. Bob went on. He knew the dog must have collided with the landing gear, so he would have to make an emergency landing and check it out. The most important thing to do before making the emergency landing was to make the plane as light as possible. The building materials for Dos Rios would have to go. Bob banked to the right of the airstrip, and while keeping one hand on the control wheel, he managed to maneuver the kitchen sink to the plane's doorway, where he shoved it out. Next went two sacks of cement, several boxes of groceries, and a fifteen-gallon can of kerosene. Thankfully, he had taken the door off the plane before he left, making one less obstacle to overcome in ditching his cargo.

Nate nodded in understanding. Bob had done just what he would have done under the circumstances. "How was the landing?" he asked.

Bob explained how he brought the Piper Pacer around for a landing. He slowed it down as much as possible as he approached the end of the runway. The undercarriage of a plane is very strong and built to handle landing on rough surfaces if need be, so Bob figured a collision with a dog probably hadn't done much damage. As he approached the end of the runway, though, he realized he must have figured wrong. His wife and a number of students from the Berean Bible Institute were pointing furiously at the right side of his landing gear. Bob knew something was wrong with it, and he worked his controls gently to make sure he got the left wheel of the plane down first. The left wheel ran along the runway, and Bob waited for the right wheel to connect with the ground. It didn't. The Piper Pacer just got lower on the right side until the end of the wing clipped the ground and dragged along the runway. Before coming to a halt, the whole plane skewed sideways in a shower of sparks from the wing rubbing on the ground. Fortunately, Bob was not hurt, which was more than could be said for the plane. The collision had ripped the right landing gear completely off, and the crash landing had bent the propeller and torn up the end of the right wing. But it was all fixable, and the Piper Pacer would fly over the jungle again.

Nate was soon in the hangar inspecting the damage. The Pacer would take a bit of fixing, but compared to the Waco biplane repair job in Mexico, this job would be simple and straightforward. Nate had all the equipment he needed and the correct blueprints for the Pacer. Fortunately, MAF now had two planes based at Shell Mera, so the pilots wouldn't be out of action while the plane was being fixed, and missionaries wouldn't have to resort to walking the jungle trails to get where they wanted to go, as they'd had to do after Nate crashed the Stinson in Quito.

A couple of weeks later, Marj and the children finally arrived back at Shell Mera, and the Wittigs returned to the United States. Soon life for the Saints was busier than ever. While back in the United States, Nate had drawn up plans to enlarge the house. It was too small for the number of visitors who flowed through, and Marj needed a separate radio room. The plans called for pushing out both ends of the house and raising the roof for a second story. This would give the home eleven bedrooms, which sounds like a lot of rooms, but it wasn't long after the renovations were complete that the bedrooms were often filled with missionaries and their guests, who stayed over on their way in and out of their jungle stations or came to Shell Mera to visit the doctor. Sometimes the rooms housed children on their way home from boarding school in Quito.

Besides enlarging his own house, Nate had to build a house for the second couple that MAF was sending to join them. The days were busy for Nate, because he also had his regular rounds of the missionary stations to make by plane. But since his furlough in the United States, he had a lot more energy, and he worked away quickly and happily. Still, he was glad when the Keenans finally arrived at Shell Mera to help with the work.

Johnny and Ruth Keenan were the perfect couple to work with Nate and Marj. They were hard workers, and they could see what needed to be done without being told. They had twin boys who were five years old, a year older than Kathy Saint. Ruth home-schooled her two boys and Kathy. She also had all the guests who stayed at Shell Merita over for one meal a day so that Marj didn't have to cook as often and was able to spend time alone with her family.

Ruth also helped with buying and packaging the groceries for the various mission stations. Marj took her to the "store" at Shell Mera, where a

Quichua Indian woman stocked the shelves from a once-a-week trip to the market at Ambato. It was best to visit the store the day after the woman's trip to Ambato to ensure the vegetables were as fresh as they could be. Otherwise, by the end of the week, everything in the store was a little wilted.

With their supplies in hand, Marj and Ruth looked at the list showing the number of people at each mission station, plus any guests they were expecting, and figured out how much fruit, vegetables, flour, rice, oil, and milk powder they would need. On the dining room table in Marj's kitchen they would separate the food into family lots and label and weigh each box for Nate to load up and deliver the next day. Marj would enter the cost of each family's groceries into a black ledger and then bill each family at the end of the month.

Johnny Keenan was an excellent pilot, and it didn't take him long to learn the art of jungle flying. Like Nate, Johnny wasn't a man to take any chances, so the two of them got along well.

It took only a couple of weeks for Nate and Marj to wonder how they'd ever managed without the Keenans to help them. Together they were responsible for serving twenty-seven missionary families. That was a big increase from the six families Nate had started out serving in 1948. And more stations were being established in the jungle all the time.

About this time, Nate got a letter from Rachel, who was back working among the Shapras Indian tribe in Peru. Rachel wrote about her conversations with Chief Tariri of the Shapras and her attempts to convince him that head-hunting was wrong. But he didn't seem to listen to what she said. Still, the two of them had become good friends. Rachel had also kept busy with her two Wycliffe coworkers translating the New Testament into the Shapras language. In the letter, she also told Nate that she couldn't shake the feeling that the Aucas were the group God had singled out for her to work with, although she didn't know how this would come about. In the meantime, she continued to trust God.

Amazingly, things began to work out, though perhaps not as quickly as Rachel would have liked. At a Wycliffe Bible Translators meeting in Peru, Cameron Townsend, the founder of the mission, announced that Wycliffe had been invited by Ecuador's president, Velazco Ibarra, to begin working in his country. Ibarra realized that someone had to help the Stone Age tribes who lived in the jungle of the Oriente to enter the twentieth century. Christian missionaries, the president noted, seemed to be the only ones who were brave enough to try!

By February 1955, Rachel was back at Shell Mera. Her first priority was to see Nate and Marj's new baby boy, Philip, who had been born right after Christmas. Big sister Kathy eagerly showed her Aunt Rachel exactly where Philip slept and how her mother bathed him.

Rachel had come from Quito where, along with a group of Wycliffe Bible Translators, she had met with President Ibarra. Nate and Marj wanted to hear all about the meeting. Rachel began by describing what she'd worn to the meeting. Since she didn't have any fashionable new clothes, she decided to wear the red headdress Chief Tariri had given her as a farewell gift. She sewed a black veil onto the front of the headdress, which, according to her, looked very glamorous in its own special way.

Nate smiled to himself. The sight of his stocky, middle-aged older sister in an Indian headdress with a veil at an official function was something he would have loved to have seen.

Anyway, Rachel's "hat" had caught the president's attention, and he stopped to talk to her. He asked her where she was going to work. "Among the Aucas," she had told him. Stunned by her response, President Ibarra had replied, "You are going to work with the Aucas? When I flew over their territory a while back, they threw spears at my plane. No white person has ever been able to live among them. Are you sure you really want to try?"

Rachel grinned at Nate. "I don't know what came over me," she said. "I forgot he was the president. I looked him right in the eye and said, 'Yes, I believe God will make a way for me to do that.'"

Nate patted her on the back. That was his sister, never beating around the bush when she had something to say. He was proud to have her in Ecuador and know that when she finally made it into Auca territory, he would be the one serving her in his plane. Of course, a lot of changes would have to take place before it was safe for a single woman to live among the Aucas. But if Rachel believed that's where God was leading her, then Nate and Marj would believe right along with her.

Within days, Rachel had her first assignment. An Auca girl named Dayuma had been located at a large plantation, called Hacienda Ila, to the west of Auca country. Dayuma had fled from the jungle after her father had been killed by another tribal member. She was too scared to return to her people, so for eight years she had been chopping sugar cane and digging yucca root on the plantation. The owner of the hacienda, Don Carlos Sevilla, a tall man about sixty years old, had allowed Dayuma to stay and work, even though he'd had some bad experiences with other members of her tribe. He bore six scars, made by razor-sharp Auca spears, that were a reminder to him of one particular rubber expedition up the Curaray River into Auca territory.

Rachel was thrilled by the way things were working out. She did not need to go into the jungle to learn the Auca language. Dayuma had come out from the jungle. Rachel was also thankful for the kindness of Señor Sevilla, who offered her the run of his house. During the day, Rachel organized her language learning and translation work, and her evenings were spent with Dayuma. It was a perfect arrangement, and one day, she hoped not too long in the future, Rachel would trek into Auca territory to meet and speak with these mysterious people face-to-face. At least, that was *her* plan.

Meanwhile, back at Shell Mera, Nate had a challenge of his own. A missionary couple were planning to move to the abandoned Shell Oil exploration base at Arajuno, and Nate had offered to help them get set up there. It would also be the closest he'd ever been to Auca territory.

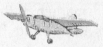

Chapter 11

Ruins of Arajuno

In early 1955, Nate touched down the wheels of the Piper Cruiser on the overgrown airstrip at Arajuno. Ed McCully sat in the seat beside Nate, his six-foot-two-inch frame slightly hunched over. Ed strained for a first look at his new home. Arajuno was an abandoned Shell Oil exploration base near a large Quichua Indian village. Like all Shell Oil bases, including Shell Mera, Arajuno had a wonderful packed sand airstrip. It was overgrown with weeds at present, but it could easily be reclaimed. That was more than could be said for the buildings. Arajuno was a ghost town. Once there had been brick houses boasting running water and electricity, as well as a tennis court, a bakery, a narrow gauge railroad, even a hotel. But Shell had abandoned

Arajuno in 1949, and by now most of the buildings had rotted away, and a blanket of vines and creepers draped over everything that hadn't rotted.

As Nate poked around the abandoned site, it made him think of his childhood. He and his brothers would have had a wonderful time exploring something like this. Maybe they would even have gotten the narrow gauge railroad working again. After prodding around for a while, Nate turned his attention back to Ed.

Ed and his wife, Marilou, had a lot of work ahead of them building a house from the ruins of Arajuno for themselves and their two small children. But Nate, intrigued by the adventure of rebuilding a ghost town, was already busy thinking about which of the old foundations would be best to use for the McCullys' new home. Of course, mixed with the adventure was the sobering knowledge that Arajuno was on the Auca side of the river, just outside Auca territory. Ed and Marilou planned to work with the local Quichua Indians on the other side of the river. One day, though, they hoped they would be able to make contact with the Aucas: friendly contact, that is.

Shell Oil Company workers at Arajuno had had some "unfriendly" contact with the Aucas. Two years before Arajuno was abandoned by Shell, three workers were killed there by Auca warriors. Two of them were Quichua Indian workers, and the third was a European man. The workers had been ambushed near the settlement and speared to death. After that it became difficult for Shell to find Quichua workers willing to cross the river from their village to work in Arajuno. A year later, the Aucas attacked again. This time they speared eight workers to death. Not surprisingly, it became almost impossible for Shell to attract any Indian workers to Arajuno after that, and so the decision was made to pull out and close the base.

As Nate and Ed worked on the new house, they never forgot they were at the edge of Auca territory. They were continually watching out for Aucas, who were easy to tell apart from the Quichuas. Although both groups were short and had jet black hair and coffee-colored skin, Quichuas wore Western style clothes, while the Aucas wore only a woven string around their waist and huge balsa wood plugs in the lobes of their ears.

Rachel had told Nate that the Aucas knew the power of the white man's gun and were afraid of it. None of the Shell Oil workers who had been killed were carrying guns. When he was alone at Arajuno, Nate worked with a small revolver tucked in his belt. At first it gave him a sense of safety, but then he began to wonder whether the Aucas would even recognize the small revolver as a firearm. It didn't look at all like a rifle, the most common gun in the jungle. Nate also wondered how safe it would keep him, since he knew he could never shoot to kill any-one, even an Auca warrior. The most he would allow himself to consider was shooting a would-be attacker in the leg, and then only as a last resort.

When the new house at Arajuno reached the roof stage, Nate decided to use a system he'd worked out when he was back in the United States on furlough. The system provided a safe way to transport lengths of aluminum sheeting on the underside of the plane. The aluminum sheets were especially useful for roofing. Nate worked out how to rig a rope sling under the plane. A partially inflated air mattress served as a buffer between the seven-foot aluminum sheets and the plane. The rope sling was tied in such a way that if one corner of it broke for any reason, the whole sling would drop off, and the aluminum sheets would drop to the ground instead of dangling dangerously under the plane's fuselage. However, anytime a pilot does something with an airplane that it's not built to do, there is risk involved. Nate was willing to take that risk himself, but he never let anyone else fly in the plane with him while he was using the sling to transport aluminum sheeting: That would be an unacceptable risk.

By mid-April, the roof was on, and all the new house needed was a few finishing touches, though not the normal touches you might think. Nate rigged up an electric fence around the yard. A powerful battery-operated light was arranged to floodlight the yard. If their dog barked, Ed or Marilou could switch the light on from inside the house. Nate also installed a very loud alarm bell that he hoped would scare off intruders.

The Quichua Indians were happy to cross the river to visit the McCullys, but they never forgot they were on the Auca side of the Arajuno River. As the sun began to set over the jungle, they would say a hasty good-bye and wade back across the river to safety, leaving the missionaries to make it through the night alone.

Each week, when he flew in groceries and Ed's *Time* magazine, Nate heard how the McCullys' mission work with the Quichuas was progressing. It was quite a while before Ed became aware that Nate had been reading his *Time* first and then carefully slipping it back into its mailing sleeve and delivering it to Ed along with his other mail. But one time Nate forgot to put the magazine back in its sleeve and delivered an empty sleeve to Ed. Nate had to confess he'd been slipping the magazines out and reading them before bringing them to Ed. After that, Ed had a running joke with Nate about him "stealing" the mail.

Marilou, who had just found out she was pregnant again, and her two toddlers often brought cookies and lemonade out to the plane where she and Ed and Nate would talk for a while. All too soon though, Nate's wristwatch alarm would sound, indicating it was time for him to be off to his next stop.

Wherever Nate flew, he took news from one missionary to another. Ed and Marilou McCully loved to hear what was happening with other missionaries, especially the Elliots and the Flemings. They all worked with the same Plymouth Brethren missionary society, called Christian Missions in Many Lands.

Jim and Betty Elliot, and their new baby, Valerie, lived twenty minutes by air north of Shell Mera at a place called Shandia. Jim and Betty were a high-energy couple who threw themselves into whatever work they had to do. The Elliots had met at Wheaton College, where Jim was an honor student and school wrestling champion.

Pete Fleming and his new wife, Olive, lived at Puyupunga, seven minutes by air southeast of Shell Mera. Pete had a master's degree in English literature and excelled in golf and basketball, two sports he didn't get to practice much in the jungle! Pete was always happiest spending his days with a sketch board and a pen teaching Quichuas to read the Bible for themselves.

There was also a large Gospel Missionary Union station at Macuma, thirty-five minutes by plane southeast of Shell Mera. Macuma station was run by longtime missionaries Frank and Marie Drown. Frank had helped Nate build the MAF house at Shell Mera, and he and Nate had become good friends. The Drowns worked with the Jivaro, an infamous head-shrinking Indian tribe. The Jivaro were called headshrinkers for a very good reason. When they killed an enemy, which was quite often, they cut off his head and shrunk it. The process they used to do this was secret, but they were more than willing to show people the results of their handiwork, which were perfectly preserved human heads, each a little larger than a baseball.

Roger and Barbara Youderian also lived at Macuma. They had been there since 1953 and helped the Drowns with their work among the Jivaro.

Nate loved to visit all of them and bring encouraging news from the other missionaries working in the Oriente.

There was one other place Nate loved to fly to as well. Unfortunately, he couldn't land there because there was no airstrip. Even so, every couple of weeks he would point the Piper Cruiser east towards Hacienda Ila. He would fly low over the main house and drop letters and goodies for Rachel. He often prayed for her as he flew. It seemed almost impossible to think that God would make a way for her to live among some of the most violent and unpredictable people on earth. But Nate knew Rachel was stubborn, and if she believed God had called her to the Aucas, she would do whatever it took to get there.

For Nate, Monday, September 19, 1955, started out like any other day. Baskets of fruit, sacks of flour, and cans of kerosene had been weighed and loaded into the Piper Cruiser. Nate fueled the plane and examined the runway. Before long he was in the air and headed for Arajuno to deliver supplies to the McCullys. It was a beautiful, clear morning, and Nate estimated visibility was about seventy-five miles in any direction. By the time he'd landed the Piper at Arajuno, he had an idea. Why not take

Ed up with him in the plane and see if they could spot an actual Auca settlement. Nate normally flew around Auca territory, but visibility was so good, it seemed a shame to waste the opportunity.

Once the supplies were unloaded, Nate suggested his plan to Ed, who also was eager to see if they could spot some of their "neighbors." Nate soon had the plane back in the air and headed east across Auca territory. Ed peered down on the sea of green trees below them. They followed a river for about fifty miles before turning north. Ed strained to see signs of life below. He saw a giant tapir sunning himself on a beach along the river. He also saw several anteaters and a flock of lime green parrots, but no sign of people. Or was there? Ed had Nate loop the plane around for another pass. Had the land below been a garden at some stage? It was hard to know, because in the jungle, within a few weeks, climbing and creeping plants swallowed up almost everything. But there was a large opening among the trees below that had probably been cleared by humans at some stage.

Nate would have liked to have stayed longer flying over the area, but he still had deliveries to make to some of the other mission stations before the day was over. It was hard to leave without having found an Auca village, but Nate finally turned the nose of the Piper westward towards Arajuno. As he did so, he thought he saw something in the distance, about five miles off the left side of the plane. He pointed it out to Ed, but Ed couldn't see

anything. Was it Nate's imagination working over-
time, or had he really seen something? He had to
check it out!

It took only a few minutes before they were over
the spot where Nate thought he'd seen something.
His heart was racing. And sure enough, there it
was, a small clearing planted with manioc and several small Auca houses. Ed and Nate whooped and
hollered with delight. They had found the Aucas.
They flew around in circles for about fifteen minutes, never going down too close to the ground for
fear of frightening the Aucas.

On the trip back to Arajuno, Nate and Ed discussed their discovery. Ed thought there must be
more than one Auca settlement, because it was a
long walk from there to Arajuno. Nate wasn't so
sure; all jungle people were good walkers. In the
end, they decided it would be best to keep their discovery secret. Who knew what might happen if the
military, the Quichuas, or the media knew the exact
whereabouts of this village.

That night, as Nate and Marj sat in their living
room and sipped lemonade, with Mt. Sangay glowing in the distance, they had a lot to talk about.
They wondered what the Aucas had thought when
they saw the plane flying overhead. What should
the next step be now that Nate and Ed had discovered the Auca encampment? Who should be
involved? Whatever happened, Nate knew he
wanted to be a part of it. Reaching a tribe that had
never heard the gospel message before and using

his airplane to do it would be like living one of the stories from the big book of missionary stories Rachel had read to him so many years ago on the roof in Huntingdon, Pennsylvania.

Chapter 12

Gifts That Weren't Spewed Up

Two weeks after he and Ed McCully had sighted the Auca village, Nate was scheduled to fly Ed, Jim Elliot, and two Quichua helpers to Villano to spend time preaching to Quichua Indians. The group had gathered at Arajuno and waited for Nate. When Nate arrived, he realized the group had more equipment than he'd thought, so he would have to make two trips. Because Villano was located on the other side of the Aucas, Nate would make a total of four trips across Auca territory. He decided he would keep his eyes peeled for more Auca settlements on each trip.

Nate flew Jim Elliot and the equipment into Villano first. He kept a sharp lookout as he flew, but he saw no more settlements. On the second trip with Ed McCully and the two Quichua helpers, Nate decided to fly a little farther to the east. The weather was clear and he was ahead of schedule, so he zigzagged the plane over the jungle valleys. About fifteen minutes out from Arajuno, they hit the jackpot! Below them were at least six Auca houses in one clearing, with smaller houses dotted around the outskirts of the clearing.

It was impossible to keep the excitement of the discovery out of their voices, and although Nate and Ed spoke in English and the Quichua helpers didn't know what they were saying, the two Quichuas were soon peering from the plane to the village below. Fear crossed their faces as they whispered the word "Auca" to each other.

Knowing that the two Quichua Indians had recognized the clearing as an Auca settlement created a problem for the missionaries. Anything could happen if the two helpers told their friends where the Auca settlement was located. Word could spread to the families of Quichua Indians who had been killed by Aucas, and they could seek revenge through a surprise attack on their enemy. That would mean the Aucas would have to kill more Quichuas in return. The bloodbath could go on for years. Somehow Ed and Nate had to convince the Quichua helpers to keep quiet about what they'd seen. As the plane taxied to a stop at the end of the Villano airstrip, Ed explained to the helpers the danger of telling their friends where the Auca village was located. They seemed to understand the importantance of saying nothing about what they'd seen, and they promised to remain quiet about it. Nate and Ed hoped they would keep their word.

Seeing the Auca village gave Nate a lot to think about as he flew back to Shell Mera alone. The Aucas were caught in a circle of violence. They killed before they listened. How could missionaries reach people who were so violent they murdered all outsiders they came in contact with? How could they get the attention of such people and, more importantly, win their trust long enough to prove they had come in peace? Nate had no answers. And he had no idea at the time that the eventual answer would involve laying down his own life to help build that bridge of trust.

On October 2, 1955, two days after Nate had dropped them off, Johnny Keenan flew back to Villano to pick up Ed McCully and Jim Elliot and take them to Arajuno. But by the time the plane reached Arajuno, the weather had turned ugly. There was a fierce crosswind blowing that whipped the trees around Arajuno from side to side. Everyone aboard the plane could see it was too dangerous to attempt a landing. There was nothing for Johnny to do but fly Ed and Jim back to Shell Mera with him and wait for better weather the next day. That night, in the Saints' living room at Shell Mera, Nate, Ed McCully, Jim Elliot, and Johnny Keenan held a "committee" meeting to talk about everything that had happened in the past couple of weeks concerning the Aucas.

They pored over maps of the area, and all agreed that seeing not one, but two Auca settlements in the previous two weeks was amazing. Maybe, they decided, God was trying to get their attention. Could now be the time He wanted them to reach out to their "neighbors"?

Marj brought them hot cocoa and homemade cookies as they continued to talk. Each of them knew that contacting the Aucas would be a difficult and dangerous task. In fact, they weren't altogether sure it could be done. Nate told the others everything Rachel had managed to find out about Auca culture from Dayuma at Señor Sevilla's hacienda. For one thing, the Auca culture was based on revenge. If a member from one tribe or family was killed, it was important for the other members of that family or tribe to kill someone from the other group. It didn't matter whether it was the person who had done the killing or a relative of the killer or someone else from the killer's group that was executed. What was important was that someone was killed in revenge. The cycle would go on and on. It was a case of kill or be killed. And it pointed out the danger the men would be in if they tried to make contact with the Aucas. To the Aucas, these men were members of the "white man's tribe" and could well be seen as targets of revenge for all the bad things white men had done to them over the past hundred years or more. Aucas had long memories when it came to revenge! It was a sobering thought, and one each of the four men present took to heart.

One of the ways to reduce their chance of being killed was to be able to communicate to the Aucas that they had come in peace. What they needed were some simple Auca phrases, and there was one Auca who could help them: Dayuma.

Jim Elliot's ears pricked up; this was a job for him. He lived only a four-hour trek from Hacienda Ila, where Dayuma was living. Not only that, but of the four men, he picked up languages the fastest. He jumped into the conversation and volunteered to go to the hacienda to learn some Auca words from Dayuma. The others agreed, and Jim Elliot had his first assignment for "Operation Auca."

The men knew that words alone wouldn't be enough to convince the Aucas they had come in peace. Before setting foot in Auca territory, they needed to demonstrate by their actions that they meant no harm. The question was how to do this. As they talked about it among themselves, they realized that giving gifts was a symbol of friendship around the world. If they gave gifts, perhaps the Aucas would understand they wanted to be friendly.

What better way to give gifts without putting themselves in danger than to drop them from an airplane. But Nate remembered a story Rachel had told him. After the three oil exploration workers were killed by the Aucas at Arajuno, Shell Oil Company had used a plane to drop gifts as a way to try to pacify them. The only problem was that the plane had overflown Auca territory, and the Aucas had thrown spears at the plane. Of course the plane was flying too high for any of the spears to actually hit it, but the Auca warriors believed they had hit and wounded it and the gifts that were being dropped from it were being vomited from the wounded plane's stomach! Nate and the other men would want the Aucas to know that they had sent the gifts and that the gifts weren't being spewed out by some wounded flying monster! The bucket drop seemed to be the answer. But would the Aucas know to catch the bucket and lift the gifts out? There had to be a way to make the bucket slide off the line when it hit the ground. Nate's first Operation Auca assignment was to devise a way to get the bucket to detach from the line so it could be left behind with the gifts in it.

It was agreed that Ed McCully would assist Nate with the bucket drop and that Johnny Keenan would free up Nate as much as possible from his regular flying duties so he could work on the project. Johnny would also serve as backup pilot for the operation if Nate was unable to do the flying for any reason.

It was after two in the morning when they finished talking about their plan and headed for bed. But even then, Nate had a hard time getting to sleep. He had two things on his mind. One was rigging the drop line so that the bucket would drop off the end when it touched the ground. The other was Rachel. Learning the Auca language and making contact with the Aucas was what she was now devoting her life to. It troubled Nate to leave her out of their group and not tell her what they were planning. He tossed and turned thinking about the situation. Finally, he decided that while Rachel may be disappointed about not being included in their plans, in the end, their making contact with the Aucas would help her to be able to live among them sooner rather than later. Besides, the men had all agreed that the fewer people who knew about their plans the better. The plan was daring and dangerous, and they didn't want others worrying about them. Nate decided that first thing in the morning he would explain it all in a letter to Rachel. He hoped he would be able to explain it to her in person after they'd made contact, but if something went wrong, he would leave the letter for Marj to give to Rachel. Finally he fell asleep.

Nate awoke the next morning thinking about broom handles. While Johnny flew Jim Elliot and Ed McCully to Arajuno, Nate began working on a bucket release system that involved using a broom handle. By the time Johnny returned to Shell Mera, Nate was ready for some trials. He had already taken the doors off the Piper Cruiser, and with a light breeze blowing from the southeast, he gunned the plane down the airstrip and took off. Johnny sat in the copilot's seat, holding a canvas bucket with rope and a broom handle attached to it.

As they circled Shell Mera, Nate explained to Johnny how the gadget should work. Johnny would drop the broom handle and the bucket over the side of the plane as they approached the target on the ground. The bucket was attached to the broom handle, and when the handle hit the ground at an angle, it would slide from the rope loops, releasing the bucket.

Marj and Ruth Keenan waited by the airstrip for the first tryout of the release system. They watched as the broom handle and bucket dangled nearer and nearer the ground. The bucket was twenty feet away, then ten; then the angled broom handle rested gently on the ground, releasing the tension on the drop line. The handle then slipped from the rope loops around it, leaving the bucket sitting in the middle of the runway. Marj gave Johnny a thumbs-up sign as he began to reel the rope back into the plane. The bucket had landed without a hitch. They tried the procedure several more times that day, and each time it worked perfectly.

It was only days later, on October 6, that Nate had enough spare time to try a gift drop over Auca territory. But what gift should they drop? It had to be eye-catching and useful. The Aucas still lived in the Stone Age; they hadn't discovered how to make metal. Nate knew if they were like the Quichua Indians, they would want metal things. Metal pots were a good choice; they were strong and didn't break like the Aucas' clay pots did. Machetes were good, too. A tree could be cut down a hundred times faster with a machete than with a stone ax.

Marj and Nate decided a small aluminum kettle with a lid should be the first gift. In it they put a dozen brightly colored buttons. Of course, they knew the Aucas wouldn't use them to button up their clothes—they didn't wear any! But Marj thought they would make nice decorations. They also wrapped some salt and put it in the kettle. Nate knew from talking with Rachel that the Aucas did not know what salt was. He decided that if he gave them some salt and they worked out that it could be used to preserve meat, it would be useful to them. Last, Marj tied fifteen lengths of colored ribbon to the handle of the kettle. She thought that ribbons fluttering from the kettle as it fell to the ground would make the kettle look like a gift.

Nate kissed Marj good-bye and gave Kathy, Stevie, and Phil each a special hug before setting out. His first stop was Arajuno to pick up Ed McCully. As before, Nate had removed the door from the right side of the Piper Cruiser to make it easier for Ed to lower the bucket to the ground. From Arajuno they headed out over Auca territory.

It took Nate only a few minutes to spot the settlement he and Ed had discovered from the air. Excitement built in the two men as Nate circled above it. Ed leaned from the plane, eager for a first glimpse of a real Auca. Spread beneath the plane was a large house made with poles and thatched with leaves. The rectangular house with rounded ends was surrounded by several tiny houses, barely big enough for a single person to stand in. The main building stood beside a stream, and the men could make out a track from the building to a small sandbar in the stream. They figured that was where the Aucas probably washed themselves and drew water. Since the sandbar was clear of any trees or long grass, Nate decided it would be a great spot to drop the bucket with the kettle in it. That way, even if no one was around to watch the drop, someone would be sure to eventually find the bucket containing the gift on the sandbar.

Nate slowed the Piper Cruiser to fifty miles per hour and started flying in tight circles while Ed uncoiled the rope and slowly lowered the bucket two thousand feet to the sandbar below. "Yes!" he yelled enthusiastically, as the bucket landed on the sandbar about a yard from the water's edge. The broom handle slipped from the rope loops as it was supposed to, leaving the bucket firmly on the ground. Ed hauled in the rope, and all the way back to Arajuno he and Nate talked about who might find the gift and what they might think of it.

Meanwhile, Jim Elliot made the four-hour trip to Hacienda Ila. Dayuma was happy to help him with a few simple words and phrases, and she didn't even ask why he wanted them. Rachel Saint was away in Quito at a conference, much to Jim's relief; he didn't want to have to explain to her why he wanted to learn the words and phrases from Dayuma.

As he traveled home to Shandia, Jim pulled the index cards he'd written the words and phrases on from his pocket and began to memorize them. "Bito weka pomopa," he repeated over and over. The phrase meant, "I want to come near you." Then he

started on "Abomiro imi?" or, "What is your name?"
And then there was the word for outsider, *cowodi.*

Back at Shandia, Jim copied out the words several times, and over the next week he gave a copy of them to each member of Operation Auca. The men all practiced the phrases and tried to imagine how and when they would get to speak them to real live Aucas in the jungle.

A week after the first gift drop, Nate and Ed returned for another drop. They thought it would be good if the Aucas got used to their coming back on a regular basis. For this drop they decided to leave a machete, which was well wrapped in canvas, since they didn't want it to swing around and hit anyone on the ground. That was, if anyone was there. All they had seen so far were Auca houses, but no live Aucas themselves.

Nate banked the plane and circled low over the house near the sandbar where they had left the kettle. The kettle was gone, as were the bucket and broom handle. Next Nate maneuvered the Piper Cruiser upstream to circle the next Auca house. They didn't want the Aucas to think they were playing favorites with one family. A canoe was resting on the bank of the stream near this house, a sure sign that someone was inside. Ed leaned as far as he could from the open doorway of the plane. All of a sudden, he yelled, "I see someone!"

As he banked around, Nate glanced through the open right side of the plane, and sure enough, two thousand feet below them was a young man running in a circle and waving his arms towards the sky. Within a minute, two other men had joined him. What could be better than dropping the bucket right where the men were. Nate banked the plane into a tighter circle over the spot and told Ed to lower the bucket, which drifted lazily from the end of the rope towards the ground. At the last minute, a wind gust blew the bucket off course, and the bucket landed in the water a few feet from shore. One of the Auca men dived right in after it. He waded over to the bucket, grabbed the machete, and began waving it wildly over his head. Ed could make out a huge grin on his face.

Over the next several weeks, Nate and Ed made a bucket drop every Thursday. After the third week, they no longer needed the broom handle system because the Aucas had become daring enough to reach for the bucket and remove the gifts inside. Nate rigged up a battery-powered loudspeaker in the plane, and sometimes Jim Elliot came along with them and spoke his Auca phrases as the bucket was lowered. The Aucas who heard his voice gazed up with wondering looks on their faces. No doubt they were trying to work out who the person above them was with the booming voice and strange accent speaking their language. They were puzzled but not frightened. They even sent gifts up to them: a headdress made from parrot feathers, a smoked monkey's tail, even a live parrot complete with half a banana to keep it occupied as it swung to and fro in the bucket on its way up to the plane.

On the eighth gift drop trip, Ed leaned out the door opening and yelled, "Bito weka pomopa" (I want to come near you). The four Auca warriors who heard him danced and raised their hands as if to say "Welcome." Nate and Ed were thrilled. The Aucas had all but invited them to visit!

This called for another Operation Auca "committee" meeting, at which Jim Elliot suggested that the time was right to land the plane somewhere near the village and wait for the Aucas to come to them. But they would need to act quickly because the rainy season was nearly upon them. He thought the next full moon, the night of January 3, 1956, would be a good time to do it, because the moonlight would give them lots of light in the jungle and make it more difficult for Auca warriors to ambush them in the dark. Nate just shook his head. Jim made it sound so easy, but in all his years flying in the Oriente, Nate had never come across a natural landing site in the jungle. He thought they'd probably have to trek in to make contact with the Aucas, and it would be better to wait until after the rainy season to do that.

They talked about the situation some more and finally it was agreed that Nate should make some more passes over Auca territory to look for possible landing sites. Nate knew it would be a miracle if he found a suitable site.

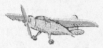

Chapter 13

Operation Auca

Nate skimmed the Piper Cruiser as close to the surface of the Curaray River as he dared. The muddy river curled below him like a sleeping snake among towering trees. Nate and Ed had just finished their ninth gift drop to the Auca village on the next river over south from the Curaray. The weather was clear and there was no wind, so instead of flying directly back to Arajuno, Nate decided to follow the twisting, brown Curaray River in the hope of finding a suitable landing spot not too far from the Auca settlement.

About four miles by air from the Auca village, or a six-hour slog by foot along a jungle trail, Nate spotted a possible landing place. It was a white sand beach perched between the jungle and the slow-moving river. He circled the plane back for a better look. It seemed promising, straight and wide, but was it long enough for a landing? Thankfully, Nate had planned ahead. He asked Ed McCully to reach into the back of the plane and grab the cardboard carton there. As Ed pulled the box into the front and lifted the lid, a puzzled look spread across his face. The box was filled with neatly stacked small paper bags, each filled with something heavy and tied shut.

Nate grinned. He loved to keep his friends guessing. Finally he explained the bags to Ed. The paper bags were filled with flour, and if they were dropped on the ground from a height, they would burst, and the flour would spill out. If Nate flew the plane at a constant speed and Ed dropped the bags at set intervals, say every two seconds, they could count how many bags fell onto the beach. Then, when he flew back to the Shell Mera airstrip and dropped the same number of bags at the same time intervals and airspeed, he could measure the distance between the first and last flour "bombs" and determine how long the beach actually was.

Ed nodded as Nate banked the Piper around for another pass over the beach. Nate slowed the plane's speed to a steady sixty miles per hour. Ed looked at the second hand on his watch. He let go of the first flour bomb bag, then a second, and a third. He had dropped five bags by the time the beach disappeared beneath them. They headed back to Shell Mera, and once again, Nate steadied the plane's speed at sixty miles per hour. Ed kept his eyes on his watch as he dropped five more flour bomb bags two seconds apart. Nate landed the plane, and he and Ed measured the distance between the first and last bags—210 yards. The beach on the Curaray River was 210 yards long. Nate whistled. It was going to be a tight squeeze landing and taking off in that distance, but it could be done. Nate would have to pay close attention to the weight in the plane though. Every extra pound of weight meant the Piper Cruiser would need another foot of landing and take-off room.

Tight as it might be to land and take off there, Nate was sure it was the best landing strip they would find. They named the strip "Palm Beach" because of the palm trees that surrounded it. Now that they had a place to land, they could make firm plans for their trip into Auca territory.

The men decided they would land, set up camp on the beach, and stay there for three days and nights. Jim Elliot volunteered to draw up plans for a simple tree house where three men could sleep in safety high above the jungle floor. He would precut all the timber so it could be put together quickly once they got to Palm Beach. Jim had some leftover scraps of wood from the new house he'd just built at Shandia. Nate would use the sling system to fly in some sheets of aluminum for a roof.

Nate was concerned about leaving the plane on the beach overnight. For one thing, if it rained heavily and the river flooded, the beach could easily be covered with water in twenty minutes, making it impossible to take off. Or worse, the plane could be washed away. It would also be impossible to protect the plane during the night. While the men were sleeping in the tree house, the Aucas could destroy the plane and leave the missionaries with no way to escape. Everyone agreed it would be best if Nate flew out each night and returned the following morning. That way he could also bring in fresh supplies.

Planning for the final stage of Operation Auca was well under way when the sun rose over the jungle on the Oriente on Christmas morning, 1955. The Saint kids were ready for action. Kathy poked Phil until he woke up, and then she hoisted him out of his crib. He had no idea what Christmas was, or even that it would be his first birthday in a few days, but Steve and Kathy needed as much help as they could to get their parents out of bed. The three of them hurried into their parents' bedroom to remind them there were presents to open. Nate smiled as three little blond heads appeared over the edge of the bed. He could remember as well as anyone the childhood lure of unopened presents. He and Marj got up, and while Nate dressed Phil, Marj made a large pan of oatmeal. With the noise in the kitchen, the rest of the household awoke.

Five other children were staying in Shell Merita. They were older children who had come down from Quito to spend Christmas with a family rather than in their dorms at school. Their own parents were missionaries who, for one reason or another, couldn't be with them for Christmas. Nate and Marj welcomed them to their home with as much love as if they were their own children. Soon the pan of oatmeal had been devoured, and it was time to open presents.

Four-year-old Steve had a pretty good idea what his present was. His dad had spent hours building a model railway complete with papier-mache landscape. The track even wound around a model of Mt. Sangay that came complete with a red light at the top and streamers that shook during "eruptions." As Nate handed the model railroad over, Steve's eyes lit up. Nate smiled. It was fun to have a son who liked the same things he had liked as a boy. It brought back memories of the B and T and P Depression Railroad he and his brothers had built as children. Nate looked forward to the many happy evenings he and Steve would spend together playing with the model railroad.

Next, Kathy opened her present. It was a doll. Kathy's six-year-old eyes widened with delight. She knew all about how to look after a baby doll, because she'd spent so much time "helping" her mother with Philip. Now they each had a baby.

Steve and Kathy never let their gifts out of their sight all day. At noon they sat down to enjoy the wonderful feast Marj had cooked for them all. Later in the afternoon, many of the young people from the Berean Bible Institute came to visit. The Saints' house was a natural gathering place for people in the area.

Because his living room was filled with people, Nate perched on the end of his bed with the typewriter in his lap, trying to finish a letter to his parents. He thought for a while about what to say regarding Operation Auca. It was a problem to him. He wasn't used to keeping secrets, so he had to be careful about what he said to his parents. He couldn't give them too many details. No one knew about their plans except the men and their wives. Aside from not wanting other missionaries to be unduly worried about the danger involved in what they were planning to do, they were afraid that if word got out about their plans, the Aucas might be swamped with photographers and journalists coming to record Stone Age men meeting twentieth-century white men.

While they needed secrecy, Nate also knew they needed prayer support, and his and Marj's parents could always be counted on for prayer during a new project. He started typing away. He wrote: "Please be in prayer for a special project the 3rd of January....We are attempting to contact a primitive group of Indians....I will be flying in support for the operation....[I] feel a real need for prayer to help at this time. A sudden move or careless word at this critical stage in the operation could slam the door of hope on people who live in the Stone Age."

The next day, Nate dropped the letter into a mail sack, and the letter began its long journey across the mountains to Quito and then on to Huntingdon, Pennsylvania. By the time it would reach its destination, Nate's parents would know far more about

Operation Auca than the letter could ever have told them.

A week later, on New Year's Day, 1956, the final plans for Operation Auca were made. With Nate no longer planning to stay overnight in Auca territory, the men felt they needed some extra partners involved in the project so there could be more than just Jim Elliot and Ed McCully left on Palm Beach. There was safety in numbers. Pete Fleming agreed to be part of the group, and Nate had also asked Roger Youderian from Macuma station to join them. This brought the number of people on the beach during the day up to five. However, because the tree house Jim Elliot had prefabricated slept only three men, and because Pete Fleming was the lightest of the team, he was chosen to fly out each night with Nate. Each day, Nate flew over Palm Beach to check whether it remained in good enough condition to land and take off on. Everything was on schedule and going according to plan.

On Tuesday, January 3, 1956, the alarm clock jarred Nate awake at six in the morning. He had managed only a couple of hours of sleep. He had spent most of the night going over in his mind take-offs and landings from Palm Beach. Nate went over every possible situation. On one landing, the plane ploughed into the jungle, and another time it flipped over after its wheels hit a stick that had gone unnoticed. Another time Nate imagined that a group of ants had tunneled under the sand as they often did, and when the Cruiser hit the unstable sand, its wheels caught in the trench and spun the plane out of control. In his mind, Nate practiced for every kind of emergency procedure he had ever heard of, hoping he wouldn't have to use any of them.

Nate also thought about the danger involved in what he was about to do. The men had done everything possible to keep themselves safe, but they had also promised each other that if Auca warriors attacked them, they would not shoot at them; they would only fire shots over their heads. There would be nothing worse than coming in peace to tell the Aucas about God's love for them and then shooting them if things didn't go as they'd planned. Each man had pledged to the others that if it came to that, he would sooner die on Palm Beach at the hands of the Aucas than risk killing people who had no idea who God was or that He loved them.

Besides, Nate and the others had already faced the possibility of death. Being a missionary in the Ecuadoran jungle was not without danger. There were poisonous and dangerous insects and animals in the jungle. Tropical diseases also posed a threat to missionaries, as did accidents from falling trees or from drowning while fording one of the many rivers that crisscrossed the Oriente. On top of that, Nate was a pilot, a job that had certain risks of its own, especially flying in the jungle. Long before he'd agreed to fly support for Operation Auca, Nate had come to terms with the fact that he might die serving as a missionary.

At 8:02 A.M., two minutes behind schedule, Nate took off from Arajuno with Ed McCully and some of the food supplies aboard. He had taken the door off the plane to enable them to transport bulky items. Fifteen minutes later, the two men were over Palm Beach. Nate swooped the Piper Cruiser down for a near landing. As wind rustled through the cabin of the plane, both men peered at the sand racing past beneath them. Were there any sticks or new holes since the last time Nate had looked? They couldn't see any, so Nate banked the Cruiser around for a landing. He set the flaps and slowed the plane as much as he could before setting his wheels down on the sand. The sand turned out to be softer than he had thought, but it was still firm enough to land and take off on. Nate cut the engine of the plane at the end of Palm Beach. He and Ed had made it safely; they were now in Auca territory. As they sat in the plane for a minute and thought about where they were, they were both filled with a mixture of excitement and apprehension about what lay ahead.

The two of them unloaded the plane. Then Nate took off to pick up Jim Elliot and the precut pieces of lumber for the tree house. Ed waited on the beach for him to return, his ears alert for the slightest sound.

It took Nate five trips to deliver all the men and the equipment to the beach. Once everyone and everything was there, they all knew what to do. Their first job was to put up the tree house so they would have a safe place to spend the nights. A nearby ironwood tree was chosen. As Ed and Jim hammered the first pieces of wood onto the tree to use as steps, they quickly realized why it was called ironwood. It took longer than they'd thought to nail steps up the tree, but no one stopped until the work was finished. Jim gave directions on how to arrange the planks of wood and pieces of iron for their tree house thirty-five feet above the ground.

Once the tree house was finished, Nate and Pete Fleming felt okay about leaving the other three men for the night. The trio would be safe in the tree house, and Nate would fly back first thing in the morning with more supplies. After all five men said a prayer together, Nate and Pete climbed aboard the yellow Piper Cruiser and took off from Palm Beach. As soon as he was airborne, Nate radioed Marj to let her know everything had gone according to schedule. It was a message she'd been anxiously waiting to hear.

Before they headed for Arajuno, Nate and Pete had one last thing they needed to do. They had to invite their "neighbors" over to visit. Nate flew over the Auca village where they had been leaving the gifts and spoke into the loudspeaker. "Come tomorrow to the Curaray River," he tried to communicate in their language. As he looked down at the faces of the Aucas, they looked puzzled. He wondered if they'd understood any of what he had just told them. Only time would tell.

The next morning, Wednesday, as soon as the fog had cleared, Nate and Pete flew back to Palm

Beach and waited for the Aucas to arrive. No one came. It was the same on Thursday. The men discussed the situation. There was no way of knowing whether or not the Aucas had understood. Maybe they didn't realize how close the men were to their village. Maybe they thought it was a trap. All the men could do was wait and pray that someone would have the courage to come and meet them.

Meanwhile, there was plenty to do around the campsite. Nate, as usual, kept a diary. This time, though, his typewriter had been too heavy to fly in, so he wrote by hand in a small pocket notebook: "Except for forty-seven billion flying insects of every sort, this place is a little paradise. With the help of smoke and repellent we are all enjoying the experience immensely. A little while ago Jim pulled in a fifteen-inch catfish. It is roasting over the fire now."

Ed had the latest edition of *Time* magazine with him. He read bits and pieces aloud to them all. President and Mrs. Eisenhower had another grandchild. Five-year-old Prince Charles of England had given his mother a painting of herself for Christmas. The head of General Motors, Harlow Curtice, was *Time*'s Man of the Year. But it all seemed a million miles away from the tiny strip of sand clinging to the side of a river on the edge of the Amazon Basin.

Every hour or so, Jim Elliot waded out into the river with his Auca phrase book. From the middle of the river he would yell words and phrases into the jungle. "We like you." "Come and visit us." "We will not hurt you." "Come and eat with us."

Each time a bush rustled or a bird squawked, the men turned to see if they had visitors, but no one came.

Chapter 14

From the Silent Jungle

On Friday morning, Pete Fleming and Nate touched down on Palm Beach at 9 A.M., just in time to join Jim, Roger, and Ed for oatmeal, which was bubbling away in a pot over the fire while Roger mixed up powdered milk to pour on it.

Nate had already had one breakfast at Arajuno, but he was always ready to eat another. After breakfast, the men took their "stations" for the morning. Nate thought it was a strange sight as he cleaned up after breakfast. Three American men were standing a few hundred yards apart, knee-deep in a muddy river yelling phrases in the Auca language. To cover as much jungle as possible with their yelling, Ed stood at the top end of the beach, Roger was near the center of it, and Jim Elliot was

171

as far downstream as was safe. "We like you. We want to be your friends. We want to come near you," rang through the jungle as the three of them yelled as loud as they could. They had yelled the phrases so often over the past few days that they'd almost forgotten why they were doing it.

As they took a breath between yells, from the silent jungle, leaves rustled. All eyes turned in the direction of the sound. Out from the thick vegetation stepped two Auca women, one who looked about sixteen years old, and the other who looked old enough to be her mother. They were both naked except for a few strands of string around their waists and huge balsa wood plugs in the lobes of their ears. The missionaries stood motionless. They were so excited some Aucas had finally arrived at their camp they almost forgot what to do next. Suddenly they remembered. In unison the three men called, "Poinani" (you're here), the Auca way of welcoming one another.

The two Auca women looked unsure of what to do next, so Jim Elliot waded cautiously across the river to them. He took both their hands and motioned them toward the campsite. They allowed themselves to be led. *So far so good*, Nate thought, as he slowly reached into his backpack and pulled out a camera.

Once the Auca women had crossed the river they seemed to relax. They squatted by the fire, and Ed offered them some lemonade. They drank it with enthusiasm. When they had finished drinking, a small, muscular Auca warrior appeared on the other side of the river. He waded across and joined the two women by the campfire. The missionaries eagerly welcomed him, and soon the three Aucas were taking turns talking as fast as they could. They didn't appear to notice that the missionaries could understand only one word in a hundred, if they were lucky.

The question of what to do next was answered by "George," the nickname the missionaries gave the Auca warrior. George trotted over to the airplane and began to climb in. His message was loud and clear: "Take me for a ride."

Nate laughed. "If that's what George wants, then that's what George will get," he said as he walked over to the plane. They found a spare shirt of Pete's and buttoned it on George, since it would be a lot cooler in the air with no doors on the plane. George was quite a sight to see sitting in the front seat of the Piper.

As the plane lifted off Palm Beach, George started yelling, and he yelled all the way to the Auca settlement. When he saw his village from the air, he yelled even louder and then collapsed into laughter when he saw the look of shock on the faces of his relatives below. Nate could not begin to imagine what the Aucas on the ground were thinking. George, who had no idea of the danger of an airplane, tried to crawl out onto the wing strut so the

Aucas below could see him. Nate was glad they'd
put a shirt on him, as it provided something to grab
onto to pull George back into the plane.

When they got back to Palm Beach, George had
a long talk with the women, and there was a lot of
giggling. "Delilah," as they dubbed the younger
woman, and the older Auca woman showed George
what they'd been up to as well. They offered him a
hamburger, complete with ketchup, which he ate
gladly. Then they handed him Ed's *Time* magazine.
George stared at it for some time, though he had no
idea of written language, photographs, or current
events.

The men passed the rest of the afternoon watching the reaction of the Aucas as they presented
them with gifts and showed them gadgets. Jim
Elliot got out a yo-yo. Nate played his harmonica.
Ed blew up several balloons, and Pete showed them
how to ping rubber bands. Roger presented them
with a skein of red wool. George took control of it
and quickly wound it around his body like a sash.
Delilah made clicking noises and smiled at his new
decoration.

Nate and Pete waited as long as they possibly
could before they flew out to Arajuno for the night.
On the way they wondered aloud what the three
Aucas would tell their fellow Aucas about the day.

As the evening wore on, the Aucas seemed
happy to stay with the remaining three men. Jim
Elliot gestured for them to spend the night sleeping
by the fire. The offer seemed to please the older

woman. However, Delilah didn't seem happy. She got up quickly and walked off into the jungle. She was gone as silently as she had arrived. George yelled after her, but she didn't turn around. After a couple of minutes, he shrugged his shoulders, stood up, and followed her into the jungle.

Jim, Ed, and Roger waited for the older woman to do the same. Surely she wouldn't think it was safe for her to stay alone with three *cowodi* (outsiders). To their surprise, she did stay, and when darkness had completely engulfed the jungle, she curled up beside the fire and went to sleep.

As the three missionaries climbed the ironwood tree to bed, they were thrilled with how the day had gone. They had made friendly contact with the Aucas. Surely, they thought, the three Aucas would go back to their village and tell the others there was nothing to be afraid of, and the rest of the village would come to visit them on Palm Beach.

What the Operation Auca men had no way of knowing at the time was why George and Delilah had come to their campsite in the first place. George and Delilah had wanted to marry, but Delilah's family did not like George and would not give them permission to marry. This had upset Delilah, who had told her family she would run away to the cowodi (outsiders) if they didn't change their minds about the wedding. Instead, her family laughed at her, so in a rage she had set off through the jungle. George followed her, but in Auca culture it is a very bad thing for an unmarried man and woman to be alone together, so the older woman had followed them to be their chaperone. They had all arrived at Palm Beach together, just as Delilah's desire to run away had petered out. They went ahead with a visit anyway. And they had an interesting time with the cowodi, who turned out to be a strange bunch but not dangerous. However, when first Delilah and then George left the campsite, the older woman had had enough of chasing after them. So she stayed on the beach and got a good night's sleep. In the morning, this created a problem for George, because he and Delilah had spent the night alone together. He had to think of a good excuse quickly. And he did. He decided to tell a lie: a lie that would change the course of countless lives.

The next morning when Jim, Roger, and Ed climbed down from their tree house, the embers of the fire where the older woman had slept were still warm. They realized she must have stayed all night and fed the fire. But now she was nowhere to be seen.

All day Saturday, the men waited for something to happen. Nate estimated it would take George and Delilah about six hours to walk back to the Auca village, if that was where they were headed. It would take them an hour or two to explain to the other Aucas what had happened when they visited the cowodi, and then another six hours for a larger group to trek back to Palm Beach. But they did not come, and by three in the afternoon, Nate felt it was time for him and Pete to head back to Arajuno.

First, though, he gathered up all the film from the cameras and letters the men had written to their wives. Whatever happened, they wanted the outside world to have a record of what they had done on Palm Beach.

As they flew back, Nate and Pete couldn't help but be a little disappointed. Why hadn't the Aucas come back? After a good night's sleep, Nate felt a lot more hopeful. Something told him today was going to be a special day.

On the way back to Palm Beach, Nate circled the Auca settlement to see whether there was any unusual activity going on. But there wasn't even any of the usual activity. The place seemed deserted. It was a great sign. Nate and Pete grinned at each other. Maybe the whole village was on its way down to the beach to meet them!

Nate slowed the plane to about sixty-five miles per hour and skimmed along close above the thick vegetation. It was impossible to spot the Aucas through the dense canopy of trees, but Nate had to try. Pete strained his eyes trying to peer through the treetops. Then, amazingly, they saw them! Wading across a stream ahead were ten Aucas headed toward Palm Beach. Today really was the day when they would meet the whole Auca village!

As the two men flew on to Palm Beach, Nate checked his watch. It was 12:30 P.M., time to call Marj on the radio and let her know how things were going. How excited she would be to know things were finally moving ahead. Nate told her they were expecting an Auca visit in the early afternoon and that he would report in with her at 4:30, though he knew she wouldn't leave the radio room all afternoon, just in case they needed help.

As the Piper Cruiser's wheels touched down on the sand of Palm Beach, Nate yelled to the others. "This is it, guys! They're on their way."

The men all let out a whoop of excitement. Their faith and patience were finally about to be rewarded.

Chapter 15

The Radio
Remained Silent

The ten Aucas creeping silently through the jungle had been up all night, carving and sharpening new nine-foot spears. *What else could they do?* they had asked themselves as they worked. An enemy had entered their territory, an enemy who had already attacked three of their people. Nankiwi had told them so. As he ran his fingers over the red wool wound around his waist, Nankiwi had told them how they had fled in panic. He and Gimari had run in the same direction, and Mintaka, who had already crossed the river, ran in another direction. Thus, the three of them had become separated, and Nankiwi and Gimari had been forced to spend the night together. But as Nankiwi explained, that point wasn't important. What was important was that a group of dangerous cowodi had invaded their territory intent on harming them just like all the other cowodi had done in the past.

This was bad news. The Waorani (the name the Aucas called themselves) had hoped the cowodi in the yellow wood-bee (airplane) might be friendly. After all, the wood-bee that buzzed over the village had dropped many ax heads, machetes, and iron pots. This was not the work of an enemy, or was it? Only a very clever enemy would pretend to be friendly and then attack. These cowodi must be extra clever!

After Nankiwi had told them all about how the cowodi had attacked them, Gikita, the old man of the village, began to recall all the awful things other cowodi had done to them throughout the years.

Through the night, Gikita told them story after story about the treacherous cowodi. He told of cowodi with guns that killed a person with a cloud of smoke, of cowodi who had stolen their children to work on haciendas, cowodi who had killed the fish and animals, and cowodi who had cleared away huge patches of the jungle. With each new story, hatred of the cowodi grew, and the solution became more clear. The cowodi on the banks of the Curaray River were surely no different from any other cowodi, and they would have to be killed.

Gikita's stories had made them all so angry at the cowodi they had forgotten to ask Nankiwi who had given him the red wool he now wore around his body as a sash or why, if the cowodi were so dangerous, had they taken him in their wood-bee and brought him back? They were questions that seemed unimportant to ask. They had already decided what to do. They would follow the old ways and kill the intruders.

The attack party had set out through the jungle with their spears. Now the sound of water rushing over stones told them they were near the Curaray. The five young men and their leader peered out from the leaves. They were on the same side of the river as the missionaries. They could see the yellow wood-bee standing at the end of the beach. They counted the cowodi; there were five of them. The cowodi were big men, and they surely had guns. The young warriors crept back from the edge of the river about a hundred yards and began to argue. They told Gikita it wasn't possible to kill five big strong cowodi who had guns. They wanted to watch the cowodi for a while. Gikita argued with them. Weren't they strong enough to kill the cowodi and protect their families and territory? Didn't they know the cowodi would kill all the Waorani if they didn't kill them first? Hadn't they listened to Nankiwi? The young men hung their heads in shame. They must kill or be killed. Now was not the time to be a coward.

Gikita announced the plan of attack. Three of the women in the party would enter the river from the far side to distract the cowodi. While their attention was distracted, Gikita would attack. He would spear each of the men himself, and the young warriors would then finish them off. They all agreed with his plan.

The women waded into the river and approached the beach from the opposite bank. Jim Elliot and Pete Fleming waded into the river to greet them, just as they had done three days before when the other three visitors had arrived.

At the same time, Gikita crept around through the jungle behind Nate, Roger Youderian, and Ed McCully. As he did so, he slipped on a wet log and fell. His spears clattered to the ground. All three men turned to see what the noise was. The four youngest attackers started to run away. They had lost the element of surprise, the most important thing in any successful attack. Still, Gikita had to show the young warriors how to act strong. With a warlike yell to the younger warriors to follow him, Gikita charged out onto the beach to begin the attack. His first target was the wood-bee pilot. He drew back his powerful right arm and hurled his first spear. It hit its mark. Nate fell onto the sand, his arm crashing against a rock, shattering the glass of his wristwatch. The hands on the watch stuck at 3:10.

Ed ran over to help Nate, and as he did so, he too felt the painful impact of a spear in his back. Roger, standing slightly back from the scene, watched in horror. As he turned his head away, he saw another Auca warrior sprinting across the beach towards Jim and Pete, who were crossing the river. With a single action, Nampa thrust his spear into Jim Elliot.

At the same time, Pete, who had been standing beside Jim, raced over to a log, which he climbed on and began to yell in the Auca language as best he could, "We just came to meet you. We aren't going to hurt you. Why are you killing us?" His question was answered with a wild cry as a nine-foot spear pierced his body.

At that moment, Roger, a veteran World War II paratrooper, knew what he had to do: He had to get to the radio. He sprinted to the plane and climbed partway into the front seat. He grabbed for the radio microphone that hung on the instrument panel. Marj would be standing by, if he could just get through to her. But he couldn't. Nimonga crept up behind him. He was puzzled by this cowodi. What was he doing? Nimonga watched as the cowodi reached down and picked up a black fruit with a vine tied to it. Nimonga couldn't understand why a man who was about to die would reach for something to eat. Still, there was no door on the plane, and this man was an easy target. The black radio microphone dangled uselessly as Roger fell from the door of the plane and landed with a heavy thud on the wet sand.

Later, as the Waorani dragged the five bodies into the river, they talked among themselves. The cowodi had guns. In fact, the gun that belonged to the man speared in the river had gone off during the struggle and grazed one of the women hiding in the jungle. Why hadn't they used their guns to defend themselves? They discussed this all the way back to the village, but they had no answer.

Back at Shell Mera, it was 4:30 P.M. Marj Saint strained to hear even the faintest crackle of a message on the radio, but there was nothing. She checked her watch. She told herself it may be a few minutes fast, though she knew it wasn't. Nate was never late for a call in, but these were special circumstances. He could be in the middle of a conversation with a group of Aucas. The thought comforted Marj. She busied herself, sitting Phil in his highchair for an after-nap snack. As she peeled him a banana, she listened closely to the radio. Five minutes passed, then ten. Marj told herself to keep calm. The radio may not be working. She would just have to be patient.

Barbara Youderian called in from Macuma, and Betty Elliot from Shandia. Both wanted to know whether Marj had heard anything. She hadn't. Their conversations were short; they had to keep the radio frequency open for Nate to call in.

Dusk fell. Marj made macaroni soup for the children and waited for the news that the Piper Cruiser had shown up at Arajuno. But the radio remained silent. In her heart, Marj knew it was too much to believe that the radio was dead *and* that Nate had willingly stayed the night at Palm Beach with the plane. Something was terribly wrong.

Marj tossed and turned in bed that night. She thought of every possible reason why Nate had not called or why he had not flown the plane out. But nothing made any sense. Something must have happened to the men. She hoped that whatever the problem was, the men were safe. Maybe they were making their way out on foot. She refused to let herself think the worst.

At first light on Monday morning, Johnny Keenan climbed into the Piper Pacer. He hadn't slept much, either. He pulled a piece of paper from his pocket and read it. He didn't need to; he'd read it a dozen or more times already this morning. It was the neatly written coordinates and instructions on how to find Palm Beach from the air. Nate had left it with Johnny just in case he needed to look for the men.

Now Johnny was almost afraid to look for them. What would he find? He would know soon enough. As he buzzed over Palm Beach, the Piper Cruiser he'd flown himself so many times before lay on the beach. It had been completely stripped of all its outer fabric covering. A chill ran down Johnny's spine. Where were Nate and the others? Johnny peered down on the muddy water, but he could see no sign of the men. With a feeling of dread, he turned the knob on the radio. "Come in, Marj," he spoke into the microphone.

Marj was grateful to have some news. At least it explained why Nate hadn't flown out. But what should she and Johnny do now? Perhaps the men were injured out in the jungle or were fleeing from the Aucas, who had attacked the plane. She had to think of a way to get help, but how?

Amazingly, almost unbelievably, there was a knock at the door. Marj opened it, and there stood Larry Montgomery, a pilot for Wycliffe Bible Translators. Larry greeted Marj and explained that he'd been passing through Quito when he had the strangest feeling he should get on the bus and make the thirteen-hour trip to Shell Mera. He apologized for not letting Marj know he was coming ahead of time. Quietly, she asked Larry to come in and sit down; she had something to tell him. For the first time, the story of Operation Auca tumbled out to someone not directly involved in it. Larry listened carefully, and when Marj was finished, he took charge. As it turned out, his friend General Harrison was in charge of the U.S. military for the whole Caribbean region. General Harrison was a Christian, and if Larry could get hold of him by shortwave radio, he was sure the general would help. Marj showed Larry into the radio room, and Larry sent out a message. The general's aide received it, and within half an hour, the general was on the line.

General Harrison called Air Force Major Nurnberg in Panama and ordered him to head up a military rescue team. By lunchtime, the rescue team was on its way from Panama to Shell Mera.

As the news of the unfolding events in Ecuador hit the airwaves, key people leaped into action, as if they had all rehearsed their parts many times. Shell Mera was about to be invaded.

In Washington, D.C., famous *Life* magazine photographer Cornell Capa slung his camera bag over his shoulder and headed for Washington National Airport.

In Quito, *Time* magazine foreign correspondent Jerry Hannifin, who had interviewed Nate for a story on jungle pilots only weeks before, jumped into his jeep and roared southward toward the Oriente.

In New York, two officers from Christian Missions in Many Lands, the Plymouth Brethren mission agency that Jim Elliot, Pete Fleming, and Ed McCully worked with, booked emergency flights to Quito.

In Los Angeles, MAF president Grady Parrot threw a few clothes into a suitcase and rushed to Ecuador to help find his friend Nate Saint.

Captain Sam Saint was called out from a conference meeting to take an urgent phone call. He never even returned to the meeting to collect his papers. Instead he went straight to the airport.

From all over the world, people wanted to know what had happened to the men who had gone off to meet a group of Stone Age people. What was being done to find them, and had anyone yet found any clues as to their fate?

Abe Van Der Puy, from HCJB in Quito, came down to Shell Mera. When he arrived, the MAF house was so crowded he pushed a piano stool into a corner, and it became his office. From there he wrote all the press releases and news bulletins that went out around the world updating the search.

Johnny Keenan flew out and fetched Marilou McCully, Betty Elliot, Olive Fleming, Barbara Youderian, and Rachel Saint. By Tuesday, every room in Shell Merita was full, and the Keenans and families from the Berean Bible Institute were taking the overflow.

Kathy Saint helped her mother make up the beds. As they moved from room to room, Kathy reminded herself that it was her seventh birthday, but somehow it didn't feel like it. Her daddy had been gone for two days now, and she was old enough to ask questions her mother couldn't answer.

On Wednesday January 11, more bad news arrived. Johnny Keenan had made another pass over Palm Beach. This time he'd seen two bodies from the air. They were in the water, and both were wearing khaki pants and white tee shirts. Any of the men in the group could have been wearing those clothes, so he couldn't tell whose bodies they were.

Back at the MAF house, Kathy and Steve Saint were glued to the window, watching the startling scenes. Three large military planes flew in, and a dismantled helicopter was wheeled out of one of them. Steve stared in fascination as the small helicopter was put back together. He would have loved to have asked his father to explain exactly what they were doing, and Nate would have loved to have told him, but it was not to be.

A search party was organized, and Frank Drown, who worked with Roger and Barbara Youderian, was asked to lead it. He had worked in the Oriente for twelve years, and he knew better than anyone what they were up against making it overland to Palm Beach. Roger and Nate were two of his closest friends. Dr. Art Johnston from the HCJB mission volunteered to go on the search party, as did several other missionaries in the area. They set out on Thursday morning, January 12, accompanied by thirteen Ecuadoran soldiers.

Marj spent her day tirelessly logging radio calls from military planes flying over Palm Beach and small planes from Quito flying in more helpers. Somewhere in the back of her mind, she also managed to plan dinner for the thirty or so people who were in the house by now.

Friday, January 13, 1956, was a day the men in the search party would never forget. They had spent the first night camped outside Auca territory. At dawn, they broke camp and headed into dangerous territory. They poled dugout canoes down the shallow, winding Curaray River.

About mid-morning, they met a group of Quichua Indians making their way upstream. This was surprising to Frank Drown, because they were coming from deep in the heart of their dreaded enemy's territory. As Frank talked with them, he learned why they were in Auca territory. The Quichua Indians were Christians from the village across the river at Ed McCully's mission station at Arajuno. Out of concern for their missionary, they had put together their own search party to go after him. But their news was not good. They had found Ed's body downstream from the airplane. One of the Quichuas had Ed's watch with him to give to Marilou. The Quichuas had taken off one of Ed's shoes and carried it back upstream and left it beside the remains of the airplane.

The search team poled on downstream, keeping a sharp, grim watch for any movement or sound that might be the Auca killers.

Finally, as the skies darkened with rain, the search party arrived at Palm Beach. The U.S. military helicopter brought in from Panama swooped down near them, as planned. It headed downstream a few yards and hovered. The men knew they were showing them where the first body was. They found the body caught in a tree branch and dragged it upstream. The helicopter moved on. Within an hour, the search party had recovered the bodies of four men. The bodies had been in the water too long and were now unrecognizable. Watches and wedding rings told the members of the search party who they were: Nate Saint, Jim

Elliot, Roger Youderian, and Pete Fleming. But Ed McCully's body was nowhere to be found. The river must have washed it away. However, the search party did find the shoe beside the airplane, where the Quichuas said they had left it. There was no doubt it was Ed's; he wore size 13 1/2 shoes. It also confirmed that the Quichuas had indeed seen Ed's body farther downstream, where it had been carried by the current. Now, at least Marilou McCully would be spared having to wonder whether somehow Ed had escaped and lay injured in the jungle. There was no doubt; all five men were dead.

Frank Drown climbed the ironwood tree to investigate the tree house, hoping to find some clues as to what had happened to provoke the horrible scene below. But there were none to be found.

The skies darkened as a fierce storm approached. The nervous search party worked quickly to dig a common grave under the ironwood tree. The thirteen Ecuadoran soldiers stood guard on the perimeter of Palm Beach. They faced the jungle, their fingers resting on the triggers of their guns, watching for the slightest movement of the leaves.

When the rain began to fall heavily, the search party pulled sheets of aluminum from the roof of the tree house and balanced them over their heads for shelter. There was a huge crack of thunder just as the bodies were being lowered into the common grave. Frank Drown said aloud a short prayer. He stood beside the grave, brokenhearted at the death of five faithful friends. He had no idea that one day he would be the only person able to give his grandchildren an eyewitness account of the funeral of their other grandfather.

As soon as the men were buried, the search team had its own safety to be concerned about. Carefully, alert to the crack of even a twig, the men made their way, mile by mile, out of Auca territory. Two and a half days later, they were back at Shell Mera, where six women waited to hear the final news. Five of the women wondered whether they were wives or widows. The sixth, Rachel Saint, wondered if she had lost the little brother she had helped to raise. Major Nurnberg, who had first spotted the bodies from the helicopter before landing on Palm Beach, tried to tell the women what he'd seen as gently as possible. But there was no easy way to say it; all of the men were dead. The wives were now widows, and their nine children, one of them still unborn, were fatherless.

That night, the people who knew and loved Nate Saint, Jim Elliot, Ed McCully, Roger Youderian, and Pete Fleming gathered in the living room of Shell Merita. Mt. Sangay, clearly visible in the distance, glowed red. Marilou McCully, who was ready to give birth within days, sat at the piano and began to play the melody to the hymn the men had sung with such high hopes the morning they had left for Palm Beach. Betty Elliot sang the words:

We rest on Thee, our Shield and our Defender,
We go not forth alone against the foe.
Strong in Thy strength, safe in Thy keeping tender,
We rest in the Thee, and in Thy name we go.

Frank Drown opened his well-worn Bible and read the verse: "Be ye faithful until death, and I will give you a crown of life."

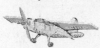

Chapter 16

The Legacy

While Nate was deeply missed by those who knew him, and especially by Marj and the children, his death was not the end of the Auca story or of the work of MAF in the Oriente.

Marj stayed on at Shell Mera for six months after Nate's death. She faithfully manned the radio for Johnny Keenan as he continued to serve the missionaries working in the jungle. At the end of six months, Hobey Lowrance and his family arrived as permanent MAF replacements for Nate and Marj.

Marj moved from Shell Mera up to Quito, where she took over running the HCJB guest house, the same guest house she had stayed in when she first arrived in Ecuador pregnant with Kathy.

Back in Shell Mera, Johnny Keenan and Hobey Lowrance continued to fly over the Auca village near the Curaray River. They carried on using Nate's bucket drop system to drop gifts to the villagers. Oddly enough, the Aucas still accepted the gifts, and even returned gifts of their own. Sometimes as he flew over their territory, Johnny would catch a glimpse of bright yellow strips of fabric decorating rooftops. The fabric was from Nate's Piper Cruiser.

Meanwhile, on Palm Beach, the remains of the Piper Cruiser sank into the mud beside the Curaray River and was soon completely covered.

Rachel Saint continued her work learning the Auca language from Dayuma, who, in the process, became the first Auca Christian. Together, Dayuma and Rachel prayed that God would open up a way for the two of them to bring the gospel message to the rest of Dayuma's people.

In 1958, two years after the deaths at Palm Beach, two Auca women, Mankamu and Mintaka (the older woman who had come with George and Delilah to visit the missionaries at Palm Beach), walked out of the jungle. With hand gestures, they made the Quichua Indians understand they wanted to make contact with white people. The Quichuas took them to Elisabeth Elliot, who was still a missionary in the area.

Eventually Mankamu and Mintaka invited Rachel Saint and Elisabeth Elliot and Dayuma to return with them to their village and live. Rachel and Elisabeth and Dayuma accepted the invitation and were welcomed into the tribe. Of course, there were those members of the tribe who were suspicious of the two women. They wondered why no one had ever tried to avenge the deaths of the five men. Perhaps the two women had come to spy on them and tell other cowodi where to find them and kill them. Dayuma, Rachel, and Elisabeth tried to calm their fears. They told them they had come in peace and that there was another way besides killing to deal with what had happened at Palm Beach. Slowly, as the three women lived among the Auca, the fog of generations of hatred and killing began to lift, and many in the tribe came to understand there would be no revenge for the killings. A new concept, one which they had no word for in their language, began to take root in their hearts. That concept was forgiveness.

In 1961, Rachel and Elisabeth watched as the first group of Waorani (Auca) Christians was baptized by Dr. Ev. Fuller from the mission hospital at Shell Mera. Shortly afterwards, Elisabeth Elliot returned to live in the United States. Rachel remained in Ecuador and lived among the Waorani for the rest of her life. She died in 1994. Thirty-eight years after her brother had been buried in Auca soil, Rachel, too, was buried there.

Forty-three years had passed since Nate Saint first pointed out Auca territory to Rachel and said, "Sis, those are your people." How right he had been. He never dreamed, however, that it would be his own death and the deaths of the other four men on Palm Beach that would help the Auca to understand the meaning of forgiveness and set the stage for his sister to introduce the greatest story of forgiveness ever told.

The legacy of the two Saint siblings, buried not far from each other in Auca territory, is that today approximately one out of ten Aucas is a Christian. And those believers are sharing a message with the rest of their tribe. It is the same message that Nate's death and Rachel's life among them so clearly illustrated. It is God's message of hope, love, and forgiveness.

In 1967, Marj Saint married Abe Van Der Puy, who had become the head of HBCJ in Quito. Abe's first wife died of cancer. Between the two of them, they have six children.

In 1970, Kathy Saint married Ross Drown, the son of Frank Drown, Nate's good friend who led the expedition to recover and bury the bodies of the five men at Palm Beach. And so it is that Frank and Nate share the same grandchildren, two boys, Brent and Darron, who are both graduates of the Air Force Academy. Flying seems to run in the family!

In 1994, a Waorani (Auca) man found a strange metal object in the sand beside the Curaray River. It turned out to be the remains of Nate's Piper Cruiser airplane, brought to the surface by flood waters after thirty-eight years of being buried. Steve Saint, also a pilot, organized a team to recover the remains, which now stand at MAF's headquarters in Redlands, California, as a silent witness to early missionary aviation.

That same year, Steve Saint helped the Waorani bury his Aunt Rachel. After the funeral, Waorani Christians asked him to come and take Rachel's place. At first the idea seemed laughable. Steve had a wife, four teenage children, and a business to run in Florida. But as he prayed, he stopped laughing and started packing. God had called him, like He had called his parents and his aunt before him, to the Ecuadoran jungle.

In 1995, Steve, his wife Ginny, and their four children moved to Ecuador to live among the Waorani. Together they are looking for ways to enable the Waorani to take responsibility for the spiritual and physical needs of the tribe so they can protect their territory, identity, and way of life. With Steve's help and encouragement, they have carved a tribal center from the virgin jungle and built an airstrip, a medical and dental clinic, and a school. The growing Waorani church is playing an important role in the development of their tribe. Members of the church are building a small airplane, which they will use to transport patients and medicine to and from the clinic and take church elders to share the gospel message in those Waorani villages that have not yet heard it. Nate Saint would have been pleased.

Elliot, Elisabeth. *Through Gates of Splendor.* Tyndale House Publishers, 1981.

Hitt, Russell T. *Jungle Pilot.* Discovery House Publishers, 1997.

Wallis, Ethel Emily. *Dayuma: Life Under Waorani Spears.* YWAM Publishing, 1996.

Janet and Geoff Benge are a husband and wife writing team with more than thirty years of writing experience. Janet is a former elementary school teacher. Geoff holds a degree in history. Originally from New Zealand, the Benges spent ten years serving with Youth With A Mission. They have two daughters, Laura and Shannon, and an adopted son, Lito. They make their home in the Orlando, Florida, area.

CHRISTIAN HEROES: THEN & NOW are available in paperback, e-book, and audiobook formats, with more coming soon!

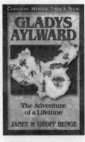
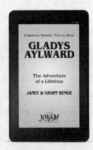
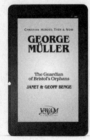
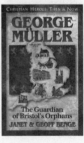
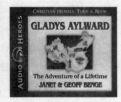
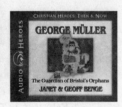

Also from Janet and Geoff Benge...

More adventure-filled biographies for ages 10 to 100!

Christian Heroes: Then and Now

D. L. Moody: Bringing Souls to Christ • 978-1-57658-552-8
Paul Brand: Helping Hands • 978-1-57658-536-8
Dietrich Bonhoeffer: In the Midst of Wickedness • 978-1-57658-713-3
Francis Asbury: Circuit Rider • 978-1-57658-737-9
Samuel Zwemer: The Burden of Arabia • 978-1-57658-738-6
Klaus-Dieter John: Hope in the Land of the Incas • 978-1-57658-826-2
Mildred Cable: Through the Jade Gate • 978-1-57658-886-4
John Flynn: Into the Never Never • 978-1-57658-898-7

Heroes of History

Available in paperback, e-book, and audiobook formats.
Unit Study Curriculum Guides are available for many biographies.
www.HeroesThenAndNow.com